First American Hospice

Three Years of Home Care

by

Sylvia A. Lack, MB BS and
Robert W. Buckingham III

In 1974, when the National Cancer Institute first made possible the inauguration of the Home Care Program of Hospice, the idea of a program for the terminally ill and their families was virtually unknown in the United States. A few Americans were aware of the highly successful experiments at St. Luke's, St. Christopher's, and St. Joseph's, and other similar facilities in England, but knowledge of their programs was limited. It took courage--and determination-- to apply the English model to the United States and to set on its way here a National Demonstration Center for services to the terminally ill and their families.

Our experience in Greater New Haven since 1974 has proved that there is a deep, unmet need in this country for services similar to those of Hospice, and that the concept is valid for meeting that need. Some 170 hospices are now in various stages of development in 39 states and the District of Columbia. All of these hospices are applying our New Haven model to their own situations.

We in Hospice are proud and honored to be in the forefront of this highly important aspect of caregiving. We are grateful to the National Cancer Institute for making this opportunity possible.

Developed under contract with the
Department of Health, Education, and
Welfare, National Cancer Institute,
Contract Number NCI-CN-55053,
September 1974 - August 1977

The Authors:

Sylvia A. Lack, M.B., B.S.   Principal
Investigator and Project Director of
the three-year contract with the
National Cancer Institute to support
the establishment and evaluation of
a program of home care.
Medical Director of Hospice, New Haven
Formerly physician at St. Christopher's and
St. Joseph's Hospices, London, England

Robert W. Buckingham III, Director of
Research and Evaluation, who carried out
the evaluation study described in Part III
of this report.
Assistant Professor of Health Education,
Teachers College, Columbia University, New
York

Contents

ACKNOWLEDGMENTS   xi

                    PART I
  HOSPICE, NEW HAVEN: SERVICES AND STRUCTURE   1

Chapter 1 Introduction   3

        2 History   9
           Groundwork . Staffing . Funding .
           Facility Planning . Chronology
           1969-1975

        3 Organization   19
           Goals and Principles . Structure

        4 Staff Training   31
           Initial Training of Multi-
           disciplinary Team . Orientation
           for Home Care Staff . Continuing
           Education for Professional Staff

        5 Volunteer Program, by Marjorie Sue   47
           Cox
           History . Policies . Recruitment
           and Training . Curriculum .
           Volunteer Assignments

        6 Procedures   75
           Patient/Family Admission .
           Procedure Manuals

Contents, continued Page

Chapter 7 Summary: Essential Features 87
of Hospice Services

PART II
HOSPICE PATIENTS AND FAMILIES: 103
A STATISTICAL PORTRAIT

8 Patient, Family, and Program 105
Characteristics
Introduction . Characteristics
of Patients and Primary Care
Persons . Utilization of
Services . Associations
Between Findings

PART III
THE EVALUATION STUDY 177

9 Terminal Care: Review of the 179
Literature
The Problem of Pain . Anxiety
and Depression . The Patient's
Family . Need for Objective
Study . Notes

10 Objectives and Methodology of 211
the Study
Objectives of Research .
Methodology . Data Analysis .
Notes

11 Findings 265

Bibliography 275

LIST OF EXHIBITS

Page

A Hospice, Inc., Organization Chart: 24
   Administration

B Hospice, Inc., Organization Chart: 26
   Medicine and Nursing

C Statistical Service Profile: Volunteers   68

D The Hospice Volunteer and the   69
   Patient/Family Record

E Statement of Policy on Insurance   72
   Coverage for Volunteers

F Excerpt from Hospice Patient/Family   81
   Record Policies and Procedures Manual

G Excerpt from Hospice Patient/Family   83
   Record Policies and Procedures Manual

LIST OF TABLES

Table   Page

1   Age of Patients   110

2   Marital Status of Patients   111

3   Number of Persons in Households of   111
      Patients

4   Ethnic Backgrounds of Patients   112

5   Socioeconomic Status of Patients   113

6   Education of Patients   114

7   Religion of Patients   114

8   When Patient Last Worked   115

9   Primary Payment Source for Medical Costs   116

10   Residence of Patients   117

11   Age of Primary Care Person   118

12   Relationship of Primary Care Person   119
      to Patient

13   Health Status of Primary Care Person   119

14   Primary Disease Site   122

15   Metastatic Site   123

16   Status upon Admission   123

17   Length of Time in Program   128

18   Number of Visits to Patients   129

19   Number of Visit Hours   129

20   Number and Types of Visits   130

21   Place of Death   131

22   Age of Patient by Primary Disease Site   134

23   Status at Admission by Primary Disease   135
      Site

24   Incidence of Pain by Primary Disease Site   136

25   Length of Stay by Primary Disease Site   137

26   Total Visit Hours per Patient by Primary   138
      Disease Site

27   Total Number of Visits per Patient by   139
      Primary Disease Site

Table		Page
28	Number of Physical Care Visits by Primary Disease Site	140
29	Number of Social Service Visits by Primary Disease Site	141
30	Place of Death by Primary Disease Site	142
31	Place of Death by Sex	145
32	Place of Death by Marital Status	146
33	Place of Death by Socioeconomic Status	147
34	Place of Death by Status at Admission	148
35	Length of Stay by Place of Death	149
36	Total Number of Visits by Place of Death	150
37	Total Visit Hours by Place of Death	151
38	Place of Death by Health of Primary Care Person	152
39	Total Number of Visits by Sex of Patient	153
40	Total Number of Visits by Socioeconomic Status	154
41	Total Number of Visits by Status at Admission	155
42	Total Number of Visits by Health of Primary Care Person	156
43	Patient Awareness of Diagnosis by Age at Admission	158
44	Patient Awareness of Diagnosis by Level of Education	159
45	Incidence of Pain by Occupation	162
46	Incidence of Pain by When Last Worked	163
47	Incidence of Pain by Socioeconomic Status	164
48	Incidence of Pain by Religion	165
49	Incidence of Pain by Whether Practicing Religion	166
50	Length of Stay by Incidence of Pain	167
51	Incidence of Pain by Place of Death	168
52	Relationship of Primary Care Person to Patient by Sex of Patient	169
53	Length of Stay by Age of Patient	170
54	Length of Stay by Sex of Patient	171
55	Length of Stay by Status at Admission	172

Table		Page
56	Summary of Hospice Staff Activities per Person per Month	174
57	Study Group: Age of Patients	232
58	Study Group: Sex of Patients	233
59	Study Group: Primary Disease Site	234
60	Study Group: Primary Disease Site by Sex of Patients	235
61	Study Group: Marital Status of Patients	236
62	Study Group: Race of Patients	237
63	Study Group: Ethnic Background of Patients	238
64	Study Group: Religion of Patients	239
65	Study Group: Educational Level of Patients	240
66	Study Group: Occupation of Patients	241
67	Study Group: Financial Status of Patients	242
68	Study Group: Hollingshead Score of Patients	243
69	Study Group: Demographic Characteristics of Primary Care Persons	244
70	Study Group: Demographic Characteristics of Patients by Primary Disease Site	248
71	Mean Scores of Psychosocial Variables for Hospice and Non-Hospice Patients and Primary Care Persons	252
72	Mean Scores of Psychosocial Variables for Patients Categorized by Primary Disease Site	254
73	Frequency of Scaled Scores of Hospice Patients	256
74	Frequency of Scaled Scores of Hospice Primary Care Persons	258
75	Summary of Differences Between Hospice and Non-Hospice Patients and Primary Care Persons on Psychological Scores as Detected by the Independent T-Test, the Paired T-Test, and the Sign Test	260

Acknowledgments

The commitment and contributions of a large cross section of our community have ensured the success of the Hospice Home Care Program in New Haven, Connecticut. Many persons involved in the development of the patient/family services are mentioned elsewhere in this report and to them, and numerous others who helped us on the way, we extend our thanks. The following deserve special recognition.

First and foremost we thank the patients and their families for the many ways in which they looked after us, thus completing the circle of team support. As representative of many, we mention the Cote, Kobylanski, Nadeau, and Gutauskas families. We thank Dr. Cicely Saunders for her inspirational leadership to the Hospice movement and Dr. James Jekyll for his guidance of the evaluation study.

Invaluable consultation to the study also came from Dr. Michael Bracken, Dr. Edward Cohart, Dr. James Collins, the Reverend David Duncombe, Dr. Daniel Freeman, Dr. Robert Hardy, Dr. Lowell Levin, Dr. Stephen Mick, Dr. Colin Murray Parkes, Dr. David Pearson, Dr. Myrna Weismann, and the members of the Hospice Evaluation and Medical Advisory Committees. Natalie Tyler performed the data collection, aided by volunteer Brian Birdwell; Elizabeth Brainard, Beverley Kelsey, Jill Phipps, Shirley Ryan, and Steve Schneider provided administrative and clerical support. In addition to the above-mentioned participants in the preparation of the report, Judy McBride, Barbara Ryan, and Jane White provided invaluable assistance in preparing the report for publication.

We thank Florence Wald and Ed and Shirley Dobihal for initiating interest in hospice care in this country. For their collaboration and encouragement, our gratitude is due to the Visiting Nurse Associations of New Haven and Branford, the Regional Visiting Nurse Association, and the Orange Public Health Nursing Association, and in particular to Betty Daubert. Similar thanks go to the Veterans Administration, St. Raphael's and Yale-New Haven Hospitals, in particular to Sara Isenberg, and to the health care community.

In addition to the National Cancer Institute, the project was supported by the Sachem and Van Amerigen Foundations, and by gifts from patients and their families. Kaiser Foundation provided a substantial grant for community relations and public information.

We thank Lawrence Burke, Project Officer, NCI, for his early recognition that there was a group of cancer patients whose needs were unaddressed and for whom continuing at-home care was required.

We are indebted to Dennis Rezendes for providing administrative and financial direction under the NCI contract. It is through his local and national vision that the program has continued to flourish after NCI. funding ceased.

Sylvia A. Lack
Robert W. Buckingham III

PART I

Hospice, New Haven:
Services and Structure

CHAPTER 1

Introduction

"Hospice" is a medieval term. It denotes a place designed for the provision of comfort and hospitality to travelers along the road. In the case of the hospice movement, the road is the course of terminal illness and the travelers are the cancer patients and the families of those patients. Hospice is a health care program that offers the kind of continuing care that enables the patient and family to live out their lives together as fully and comfortably as possible.

Since September 1974, Hospice at New Haven, Connecticut, enabled by a grant from the National Cancer Institute, has conducted a Home Care service for terminally ill patients and their families. Hospice is the first such program in the United States. Its Home Care service, tailored to meet the individual requirements of each patient and family, is directed by a full-time Hospice physician and staffed by an interdisciplinary team. The team consists of an additional physician, registered nurses, licensed practical nurses, a social worker, a clinical pharmacist, clergy, other professionals as needed, a volunteer director, volunteers, and secretaries. By utilizing such a blend of professional, nonprofessional, and volunteer skills, the staff at Hospice have developed a comprehensive, integrated, and complete care program, capable of specialized and consistent support of the patient and family.

The Hospice Home Care program aims at satisfying the psychological, physiological, spiritual, and social needs of the dying patient and the patient's family. By employing specialized and intensive medical, nursing, and pharmaceutical services, the treatment program can be directed at the patient's symptoms—pain, nausea, and other attributes of terminal disease—which deprive the patient of strength needed to participate in living. By managing these symptoms, the Home Care team endeavors to keep patients comfortable, alert, and in good spirits during their last days, reducing preoccupation with suffering and enhancing the quality of life.

Because of the disruption of family life style caused by the many changes that occur during the course of terminal illness, Hospice personnel recognize the importance of sustaining continuity of care. Terminal illness shatters the equilibrium of the family group; therefore, it is the patient and the family who are designated as the unit of care. Medical care and supportive counseling involve both the patient and family by day in their homes. The team is also on call for emergencies at night and on weekends.

A vital aspect in maintaining family cohesion is the training of a "primary care person" in nursing methods. Such training allows someone in the family to participate actively in the care of the patient. In addition, Hospice volunteer services permit the family to have more free time to draw closer to the patient and to one another. By thus incorporating the family into the patient-care system, the program reduces the patient's anguish of loneliness and isolation and improves the ability of the Hospice team to provide support for the family before and after the patient's death.

Maintenance of the family as a cohesive, supportive unit, provision for the relief of loneliness and separation anxiety, and symptom control for the maximum comfort and alertness of the dying patient are key objectives of the Hospice staff. If the needs of the patient's family are inadequately attended to, attempts at meaningful care of the patient may be in vain. Thus, consideration of the family is accepted as an essential component of Home Care. Patient's behavioral patterns often undergo a marked change, and overlapping defenses of denial and symptoms of depression dominate their relationships with others. At this time the medical personnel, and more especially the families, desperately need to understand that the patient's changed behavior is not a result of something they may or may not have done but a predictable response to a very difficult situation. Only when feelings of anger, guilt, and loneliness experienced by the family members are vented and dissipated can the unspoken sense of alienation in the dying patient be alleviated. Family problems are often too closely related to interaction with the terminally ill cancer patient to go unheeded.

Hospice is building a unique 44-bed
facility to complete the total Hospice program.
This facility is designed to supply in-patient
care and will especially aid the following kinds
of patients:
1. those who, with additional support,
    could remain at home
2. those who are unable to cope any longer
    in their own homes
3. those whose symptoms can be alleviated
    by round-the-clock attention, and then
    discharged to their homes
4. those whose families, wearied by pro-
    longed nursing, need a rest themselves
5. those whose families have been unable
    to take a vacation because of their
    nursing commitment
In endeavoring to provide the best possible
terminal care to patients and their families,
and in seeking to expand opportunities for
health care personnel to learn from close
contact with the dying and the bereaved, Hospice
is modeled after its British prototype,
St. Christopher's, which was built in London
in 1967. The Hospice philosophy, both in London
and in New Haven, emphasizes flexibility in
caring for the patient and family. Basic to
the Hospice Home Care system is the belief in
the right of the terminal patient to die at
home, if that person and the family wish,
rather than in the depersonalizing surroundings
of an acute-care hospital or nursing home.
By integrating humanistic (spiritual,
psychological, and social), medical, and
nursing care, Hospice Home Care attempts to
provide a warm atmosphere of peace and friend-
liness in which the patient can ask questions
about his or her condition and receive answers.
Hospice is concerned with teaching the health
professionals and relatives that evasion and

deception may exacerbate the patient's difficulties. Whether or not the patient accepts the imminence of death, it is essential that the staff are prepared to confront the truth about the patient's imminent death and that they listen openly and supportively to the patient as the final stages of his life and illness are resolved.

Even in its incipient stages, the comprehensive Hospice Home Care program can be seen as valuable insofar as it attains its goal of maintaining a quality of life satisfactory to both patient and family. Joan Craven and Florence Wald ("Hospice Care for Dying Patients") have stated that, "What people need most when they are dying is relief from the distressing symptoms of their disease, the security of a caring environment, sustained expert care, and the assurance they and their families won't be abandoned" by family and care-givers. It is hoped that by eliminating the problems that have been neglected or caused by existing forms of terminal care, Hospice can meet such primary needs.

Structure of the Report

This report on the first three years of the Hospice Home Care Program is presented in three major sections. The first section is a review of Hospice's history and its organizational and administrative structure. The second section contains a detailed analysis, with tables, of the characteristics of Hospice's patients and family members. The third section contains the highlights of a research study conducted to evaluate, in an objective, quantitative manner, the effects of Hospice care. Footnotes appear at the end of the chapters in which they occur.

7

CHAPTER 2

History

The hospice movement began in Great Britain. Dr. Cicely Saunders, while working at St. Joseph's Hospice in London, formulated an innovative approach to the care of the terminally ill and their families. Her leadership resulted in the establishment of St. Christopher's Hospice, a 54-bed inpatient facility. As early as 1963, Dr. Saunders had spoken at Yale University about her efforts to help the terminally ill. By the time St. Christopher's had opened its doors in 1967, a group of clergymen and medical personnel in the New Haven area had already begun to plan for the development of a similar program on this side of the Atlantic.

GROUNDWORK

In order to assess the need for a Hospice program in the Greater New Haven area, a group of health care professionals prepared a study entitled "Interdisciplinary Study for Care of Dying Patients and Their Families." Florence Wald, R.N., Research Associate at Yale University School of Nursing and its former dean, was the principal investigator. Co-investigators were Edward Dobihal, Ph.D., Director of the Department of Religious Ministry at Yale-New Haven Hospital and Clinical Associate Professor of Pastoral Theology at Yale Divinity School; Ira Goldenberg, M.D., Professor of Clinical Surgery at Yale University School of Medicine; Morris Wessel, M.D., Associate Clinical Professor of Pediatrics; and Kathryn Klaus, R.N.

The study was completed in October 1969 and a research conference was held in October of the following year.

A steering committee for the proposed Hospice program was formed in April 1971 consisting of 15 medical, pastoral, and community leaders. The following month, a meeting was held to organize task forces in the areas of finance, research, building and site selection, community relations, patient care, internal organization, and professional relations.

STAFFING

The Board of Directors of Hospice, Inc.
incorporated in November 1971. The following
summer a Personnel Committee was formed and a
(part-time) Finance Coordinator was hired.
Florence Wald and three additional persons were
employed for a combined total of two full-time
positions to plan and administer the development
efforts of the board and task forces. The
office operated out of two rooms in the Church
of the Redeemer on Cold Spring Street in New
Haven. From the start volunteers were vital to
the program, assisting with clerical tasks in
the office and functioning on Hospice task
forces. Hospice volunteers represented not only
health care workers but also people from many
backgrounds. They brought to Hospice professional expertise, knowledge of the community
and consumer needs, and educational skills.

In order to keep the public informed about
the proposed Hospice program, two Community
Relations Coordinators were hired at 50 percent
time in March 1973.

Later in that year, Dennis Rezendes was
retained as a consultant to assist the board
and staff in dealing with regulatory agencies
such as the State Commission on Hospitals and
Health Care, to help with the site selection,
and to assist in obtaining licensures. In February of 1975, Mr. Rezendes was named full-
time Hospice administrator.

A year later, the staff had expanded
to include a Coordinator of Research and
Evaluation, a Director of Development, and
a Public Information Director.

Staffing of the medical personnel evolved
gradually. In 1973 Dr. Sylvia Lack was
selected by the Hospice board to direct

the Home Care program. Dr. Lack had previously served as Medical Officer at St. Joseph's and St. Christopher's Hospices in London. Sister Mary Kaye Dunn, O.S.F., R.N., B.S., then a staff nurse dealing with advanced cancer patients at St. Mary's Hospital, affiliated with the Mayo Clinic in Rochester, Minnesota, was hired in July to work with Dr. Lack in formulating the Home Care program. They began their work in September 1973.

A core team for home care--consisting of one registered nurse, three licensed practical nurses, a social worker, and a secretary-- was hired in January 1974 and began specialized training. A director of volunteers joined the staff in April of that year.

State Approval for the Home Care program was granted in March 1974 and for the inservice service that May. At this time, the Board of Directors was selectively enlarged and a Medical Advisory Committee was established for the protection of patient/families.

FUNDING

At its first meeting on November 19, 1971, the Board of Directors of Hospice, Inc., recognized the need for substantial fund-raising efforts and made immediate applications for grant monies to the New Haven Foundation and the Connecticut Regional Medical Planning Group. Soon after, the Finance Task Force began to research the foundations that were potential supporters of the nascent program and developed an operating budget in preparation for grant applications.

Receipt of an anonymous $10,000 challenge grant during the summer of 1972 provided welcome impetus to fund-raising efforts.

By November of that year, completed grant applications had been sent to the Commonwealth Foundation and the van Ameringen Foundation.

Funds from the National Cancer Institute were received in the fall of 1974, in addition to a two-year grant from the Kaiser Foundation in the amount of $125,000 for community relations and public information.

By early 1975, support to the Home Care program was being subsidized by a 15-month, $331,762 contract with the National Cancer Institute, a two-year grant from the Sachem Fund in the amount of $100,000, and by a $78,830 van Ameringen Foundation grant.

By the end of 1976, more than $400,000 had been raised in private, corporate, and foundation subscriptions for the capital costs of the Hospice building, in addition to operational monies for the ongoing program.

Efforts in 1976-77 to secure the remaining funds for the construction of the Hospice facility from the Department of Commerce were unsuccessful. Meanwhile, however, Connecticut Governor Ella T. Grasso asked the General Assembly to appropriate $1.5 million (half the total building and equipment costs) from the state budget. A week and a half later, U. S. Representative Robert N. Giaimo (3rd District) testified before the House appropriations committee urging the federal government to match the amount allocated by the Connecticut Legislature.

These new developments at the state and federal level were coupled with steadily growing contributions from the Annual Appeal and from memorial gifts as the program became important in the area. As a result it became possible to plan for ground-breaking for the Hospice building in November 1977.

FACILITY PLANNING

Prentice & Chan, Ohlhausen was selected as the architectural firm for the Hospice inpatient facility. By April 1973, negotiations for the purchase of a site in Hamden, a suburb of New Haven, were in difficulty. We had moved too fast without educating the community on the nature and purpose of Hospice before seeking their support. As public resistance to the required zoning variance mounted, purchase of the Hamden site was abandoned and a new search begun.

A year later negotiations began for a six-acre site in Branford. This site was finally purchased in December 1975, this time with enthusiastic neighborhood involvement. In October 1975, the First National Hospice Symposium was held adjacent to the building site. Some 70 persons attended, representing more than 20 Hospice planning groups.

Prentice & Chan, Ohlhausen completed the working drawings in 1975. The plans were reviewed by the Hospice board, state officials, and members of the staff. Following a public hearing, Branford officials (including the First Selectman, the Town Engineer, the Fire Marshal, the Health Officer, and members of the Planning and Zoning Commission) reviewed and approved the floor and site plans. Ground was broken in late 1977.

14

HOSPICE, NEW HAVEN--CHRONOLOGY 1969-1975

1969	
October	Completed study of need for Hospice in New Haven.
1970	
October	Held research conference.
1971	
April	Formed steering committee.
May	Organized Task Forces in finance, research, building and site selection, community relations, patient care, internal organization, and professional relations.
November	Board of Directors incorporated and held first meeting. Made first application for grant funds and undertook program to introduce Hospice to the community at large.
1972	
February	Formulated statement of Hospice philosophy. Finance Task Force set up bookkeeping system, developed operating budget, and researched potential foundations for grant support.
Summer	Received $10,000 anonymous challenge donation. Moved to two-room office facility. Hired Finance Coordinator (25% time). Formed Personnel Committee.
August	Hired Florence Wald and three others to administer planning and development efforts of Board of Directors and Task Forces
October	Hired architects Prentice & Chan, Ohlhausen.

1972

November   Committee met with Commissioner of
Health to obtain support.
Completed grant applications to three
foundations.

1973

March   Meeting of architects for Hospice and
St. Christopher's.
Hired two Community Relations
Coordinators (half time).

April   Hired Dr. Lack and Sister Mary Kaye
Dunn to direct Home Care Program.
Hired accounting firm Ernst & Ernst,
which undertook feasibility study.
Began search for new facility
location after Hamden site failed.

October   Moved offices to present location at
765 Prospect Street, New Haven.

November   Sought separate licensure for Home
Care Program and Inpatient Program.

December   Hired consultant to assist in dealing
with regulatory agencies, in site
selection, and in obtaining
licensure.

1974

January   Hired and began training of core team
for Home Care Program: one regis-
tered nurse, three licensed
practical nurses, one social worker,
one secretary.

March   Conn. Commission on Hospitals & Health
Care approved Home Care program.
Selected first Home Care patients for
pilot study.

April   Began negotiations for Hospice site
in Branford.
Hired Director of Volunteers.

May   Public hearing held by Commission of
Hospital and Health Care.

1974

May	Certificate of Need approved for Inpatient program.
	Dr. Lack hired full time.
	Medical Advisory Committee formed.
	Agreement reached with Visiting Nurse Association.
	Accounting system established.
	Application procedure for NCI funds initiated.
Fall	Received funds from NCI.
	Received grant from Kaiser Foundation.

1975

February	Hired Dennis Rezendes full-time administrator.
	Grants for Home Care Program include contract from NCI, grants from the Sachem Fund and van Ameringen Foundation.
October	First National Hospice Symposium held, attended by representatives of more than 20 Hospice planning groups.

1976

May	Working drawings for Hospice facility completed.
October	Branford officials approved site plans after public hearing.

CHAPTER 3

Organization

The Hospice concept is so innovative that
the task of creating and staffing a structure
to deal effectively with the needs of the
terminally ill and their families was
formidable. Two fundamental difficulties
faced--and continue to confront--the New Haven
Hospice: first, the status quo for terminal
care in the American medical community, and
second, the problem of fitting Hospice into
the bureaucratic maze of American health care
without changing its purposes and nature.

Unfortunately, in the United States today
the patient with a chronic, terminal illness
is typical of that segment of the patient
population which is, on balance, harmed rather
than helped by the treatment modalities of
modern medicine. It is an ugly reality that

many patients, once a diagnosis of terminal disease is made, are relegated to that stereotyped "remote corner of the ward" to die because, it is believed, nothing more can be done to help.

Dr. Elisabeth Kubler-Ross and others have shown us that the dying do indeed have great needs that can be met, and that their families often suffer considerable emotional and physical harm during the illness and bereavement period. Others, such as Dr. Cicely Saunders of London's St. Christopher's Hospice, have demonstrated the possibilities of remarkably sensitive, efficient, economical, and comprehensive terminal care in facilities such as St. Christopher's and other British hospices.

The second problem is to sustain Hospice within the framework of American medical bureaucracy. The concept of Hospice home care cuts across many boundaries. It challenges the assumption that the hospital is invariably the best place for a sick person to recuperate--or die. It states that a trained, sensitive volunteer can often do more good than the world's best surgeon or most expensive machine. It says that even terminal cancer patients can experience life without intractable pain or drug-induced stupor.

Despite the benefits of the Hospice program to patients and families, these characteristics make Hospice care a square peg to be fitted into the round holes of Medicare, Medicaid, certification, various reimbursement plans, and physician referral systems. In addition, considerable misunderstanding and ignorance within the community itself often creates a distorted picture of Hospice.

GOALS AND PRINCIPLES

The goals of the Hospice Home Care program are as follows:

1. to ease the overall stress and burden of a traumatic life experience by sharing and working with the expressed needs-- physical, emotional, social, and spiritual-- of the cancer patient and the family

2. to aid the patient in the struggle to maintain independence and to experience death with dignity

3. to minimize the painful and damaging effects of the family's bereavement

To strengthen the bond between patients and families in need of comprehensive care, and the caregivers, administrators, and citizens who formulate and provide the appropriate services, the following principles have been developed by Hospice.

1. Comprehensive care requires interdisciplinary expertise and broad utilization of other community services. Furthermore, constant exposure to terminal situations necessitates much peer support and consultation. For the Home Care team to provide this care, decision-making must be a team effort. The Home Care "hierarchy" is therefore decentralized to allow constant interchange of ideas and suggestions, as opposed to more traditional physician-dominated decision-making.

2. Both the Home Care and the administrative bodies need persons who have had contact with other community health organizations, cancer groups, and so forth to facilitate the complex task of coordinating these many services into a therapeutic milieu

suitable to varying patient and family needs.

   3. Because dialogue with dying patients has been the real key to redesigning terminal care, the clergy and others who regularly counsel patients have played an important role in Hospice.

   4. Care-givers with previous experience in terminal settings of any kind are valued for technical expertise while lending a certain perspective and stability to the team.

STRUCTURE

Board of Directors

   Since incorporating in 1971, the Hospice board has been led by the Reverend Edward F. Dobihal, Jr., Clinical Professor of Pastoral Care, Yale Divinity School, and Director of Religious Ministries at Yale-New Haven Hospital. The rest of the board is composed of care-givers, clergy, researchers, business persons, and other private citizens, including two family members of deceased patients who had been served by Hospice Home Care. This diverse membership has produced actions based on wide knowledge of many facets of community concern. As stated in the Hospice, Inc., by-laws, the Board of Directors "shall have at least one-quarter of its membership composed of persons engaged in the healing arts, two of whom shall be a physician and dentist, one-quarter members of the community elected directly at an annual meeting...and one director shall be chosen to represent each group covered by any group service agreement hereinafter negotiated." The board has ultimate responsibility for business, property,

22

and other major affairs; the relationship
between the board and other administrative
personnel is not unlike that of many
corporations.   (See Exhibit A)

Board Committees

The board is currently aided by 13 committees, each of which reports to the board.   Among
these are the Capital Campaign Committee, which
directs capital fund-raising; the Development
Committee, which oversees financing and estab-
lishes borrowing policies; Hospice Facility
Committee, which oversees building development;
the Auditing Committee; and other committees
concerned with Hospice resources and personnel.
An important characteristic of these
committees is that each is composed of some
board members, some Hospice staff members, and
people from the community at large.   This serves
further to make Hospice, Inc., responsive to
staff and community needs

Administrator

The executor of board policy and the
initiator of innumerable other activities is the
Administrator, Dennis Rezendes.   Before joining
Hospice as full-time administrator, Mr. Rezendes
served as President of the Community Research
and Development Corporation of Hartford,
Connecticut.   His wide background in both business and city administration included acting as
consultant to numerous clients in governmental
foundations and private organizations; he also
served as president of the Greater Hartford
Process in Hartford, and vice president of the
American City Corporation of Columbia, Maryland.

Joint Conference Committee

Below the Administrator is the Joint

23

Exhibit A

HOSPICE, INC.

ORGANIZATION CHART
ADMINISTRATION

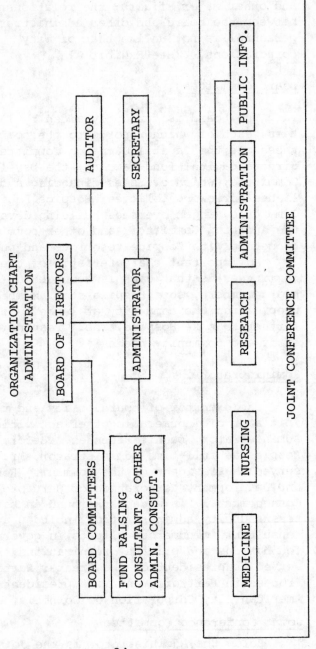

24

Conference Committee (JCC) which serves as an
important liaison between board and staff members. It is composed of representatives from
Medicine, Nursing, Research, Administration,
and Public Information. The JCC makes decisions
at the interdepartmental level in order to
recommend policy to the board and functions as
an open forum for discussion of interdepartmental conflicts and problems.

Home Care Staff

The Home Care Program is the heart of
Hospice. Under the general supervision of the
Medical Director and Home Care Program Coordinator (see Exhibit B), this interdisciplinary team
draws upon medical and nursing staff, a thoroughly trained corps of volunteers under a full-
time director, a social worker, numerous
professional consultants (most of whom provide
their time on a volunteer basis), and other
supportive staff such as secretaries.
The Home Care staff provide a range of
skills and experience essential for the
development and effective implementation of
this innovative health care concept.

Sylvia A. Lack, Medical Director (full time).
Educated at London University (M.B., B.S.) and
St. Bartholomew's Hospital, London, Dr. Lack
served as House Surgeon at Whipps Cross Hospital,
London, and House Physician in General Medicine
at the same hospital. She first became
interested in the Hospice movement in England
in 1971, when she served as Medical Officer at
St. Christopher's Hospice and St. Joseph's
Hospice, both in London. She has served as
Hospice Physician at Hospice, Inc., since
August 1973.

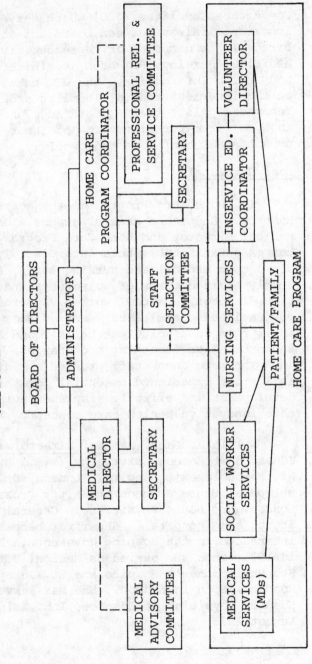

Exhibit B

HOSPICE, INC., ORGANIZATION CHART
MEDICINE AND NURSING

BOARD OF DIRECTORS

ADMINISTRATOR

MEDICAL DIRECTOR

SECRETARY

MEDICAL ADVISORY COMMITTEE

HOME CARE PROGRAM COORDINATOR

PROFESSIONAL REL. & SERVICE COMMITTEE

SECRETARY

STAFF SELECTION COMMITTEE

VOLUNTEER DIRECTOR

INSERVICE ED. COORDINATOR

NURSING SERVICES

PATIENT/FAMILY

SOCIAL WORKER SERVICES

MEDICAL SERVICES (MDs)

HOME CARE PROGRAM

Sr. Mary Kaye Dunn, RN, Home Care Program Coordinator (full time). Sr. Mary Kaye Dunn received her B.S. in Nursing at the College of St. Theresa, Winona, Minnesota. Formerly Head Nurse and Nursing Instructor at St. Mary's Hospital, Rochester, Minnesota, she was a lecturer in pastoral care and has a Yale University School of Nursing courtesy faculty appointment. Sr. Mary Kaye came to Hospice with experience gained in three years work on a leukemia ward.

William S. Norton, M.D., Associate Physician (half time). Dr. Norton graduated from Columbia Medical School. His experience includes 30 years of private practice in internal medicine. He was attending physician at, and is now a trustee of, St. Luke's Hospital Center in New York City, and is a member of their Hospice advisory committee.

Richard Glendon, M.D., Associate Physician (half time). Dr. Glendon, a family practitioner, is a graduate of Case Western Reserve University with experience establishing a new health care delivery system in group practice with the National Health Service Corps. He is also active in other innovative medical areas: a founder of New Haven Halfway House and physician for the Fair Haven Clinic, serving a poverty area.

Joni Quarberg, RN, Patient Care Coordinator (full time). Another RN diploma graduate of St. Mary's School of Nursing, Rochester, Minnesota, where she was also a member of the staff, Ms. Quarberg joined the team with two years of experience as head nurse on a leukemia ward.

<u>Charlotte Gray, R.N., Inservice Education
Coordinator (full time)</u>. Ms. Gray received her
BS in Nursing Education from Marquette
University and was an instructor in medical-
surgical nursing at Yale-New Haven Hospital.
Her training in terminal care at St. Luke's
Hospice in England provided a valuable comple-
ment to the experience of Hospice personnel who
trained at St. Christopher's.

<u>Ruth Mulhern, RN (60 percent time)</u>. A
graduate of the Hospital of St. Raphael, New
Haven, Ms. Mulhern was a surgical nurse,
evening supervisor, and service coordinator
with Homemakers-Upjohn. She is the only team
member with previous home care experience.

<u>Patti Ruot, LPN</u>. After working for two
years as a home care staff nurse, Ms. Ruot
took a maternity leave and has now joined the
staff as the Inpatient Clinical Advisor.

<u>Shirley Dobihal, LPN (60 percent time)</u>.
Ms. Dobihal worked at Yale-New Haven Hospital
and studied seven months at St. Christopher's
Hospice in London.

<u>Peter Lynch, MSW</u>. Mr. Lynch was
educated in Ireland and at the University of
Connecticut School of Social Work. He worked
at the Veterans Administration Hospital in
Newington, Connecticut. He was particularly
welcomed for his prior experience working in
home care with an interdisciplinary team.

<u>Sue Cox, Director of Volunteers</u>. Before
coming to Hospice, Ms. Cox was Program Director
of a convalescent hospital, training and super-
vising volunteers. She screens applicants and
trains and supports the volunteer staff.

Kay Barone, Admissions Registrar (full time). Formerly a secretary at Yale-New Haven Hospital before joining Hospice, Ms. Barone is now Admissions Registrar on the staff.

Father Ed Simas (20 percent time). Father Ed Simas came to Hospice from the chaplaincy at Albertus Magnus College. A recent addition to the team, he is concentrating on four areas of pastoral care: direct patient-family care; coordination and education of community clergy; assessment of total pastoral care needs; and staff support.

Other clergy. Pastoral care has always been a part of the Hospice concept; these services are ordinarily provided by the priest, minister, or rabbi in whose congregation the patient/family resides. Hospice also has among its board of directors and task forces members of clergy who have volunteered their services.

Consultants. Other community-based health providers advise the Home Care team on a consultant basis. The essential feature of all Hospice Home Care consultants is that they are willing to do home visits and are able to function in the home setting away from their usual setting with equipment, tests, and ancillary help at hand. The consultants on call during the first three years of the Home Care program are shown below.
  James Collins, M.D., Physician Consultant in Radiation Therapy
  Frederick Earl Dugdale, M.D., Consultant in Physical Medicine
  Len Farber, M.D., Physician Consultant in Oncology

Selby Jacobs, M.D., Consulting Psychiatrist

Arthur G. Lipman, Pharm. D., Clinical Pharmacist Consultant

David Melchinger, M.D., Physician Consultant in Internal Medicine

James Nordlund, M.D., Physician Consultant in Dermatology

Sherwin Nuland, M.D., Physician Consultant in Surgery

Margaret Renfro, RPT, Physical Therapist

Morris Wessel, M.D., Physician Consultant in Pediatrics

CHAPTER 4

Staff Training

The interdisciplinary continuing care team
at Hospice, New Haven, will serve as a model in
its approach to the care of the terminally ill.
Therefore, one of the major objectives in
structuring Hospice was to develop, provide,
and evaluate an interdisciplinary educational
program for health care specialists. The multidisciplinary home care team trained during the
1974-77 period was the core staff who will
assist in educating the full complement of the
Hospice team when the building opens. The team
consists of physicians, nurses (R.N.s and
L.P.N.s), a pharmacist, psychiatrist, physical
therapist, social worker, volunteer director and
volunteers, and secretaries.

The extent to which terminal cancer and its
treatment has profound and far-reaching effects
for the patient and his or her nearest relatives

is now being recognized. Health care specialists and planners alike are beginning to address these physical, spiritual, and psychosocial problems, as evidenced by the increasing number of courses and workshops dealing with death and dying. The Hospice education program for health care specialists has offered valuable clinical practice in addition to the theoretical examinations of the subject in workshops. The coordinated and cooperative effort of the team in providing continuing care services on an at-home basis to patients whose cancer will not be controlled or cured (and their families) has made it possible for those with advanced disease to be comfortable, alert, and free to experience life more meaningfully, while remaining in the atmosphere of their home for as long as appropriate.

Because the attitudes of others are important in the patient's adjustment to illness and its treatment, the plan of care evolves around the family as a unit. The patient and the family receive supportive guidance and instruction in self-care. Following the death supportive services are also available to surviving family members. These concepts actively guided the design of the educational program for health care specialists.

First, a six-week training program was developed for the multidisciplinary continuing care team (core staff). Later a six-week training program was implemented for core staff members who were to be hired during the second and third years of the project. To keep the team abreast of recent advances in cancer care, a bimonthly educational program for the professional staff was established. Separate training programs were designed for the bereavement follow-up team and the community based volunteers. These various training programs are described below.

Initial Training of the Multidisciplinary Team

Objectives. The six-week training program for the continuing care team was designed so that each team member would:

1. become knowledgeable about Hospice's philosophy and goals as evidenced in its history and current activities
2. learn the rationale and therapeutics employed in the application of Hospice principles of patient/family care
3. receive opportunities for learning and demonstration of patient/family care skills in an interdisciplinary setting
4. be introduced to, and participate in, the behavioral dynamics of a team
5. become knowledgeable about Hospice policies and procedures
6. receive an opportunity to demonstrate patient/family care skills in the home setting
7. become knowledgeable about the health care delivery systems and resources in the local community

Program. To achieve the first objective--knowledge of Hospice philosophy and goals--team members were required to attend a Hospice open forum and conferences with staff, the Board of Directors, and/or Task Force members (minimum of five sessions, total 2 1/2 hours.) Audiovisual presentations including slides and films on St. Christopher's Hospice and such topics as control of terminal pain and care of the family were scheduled (total 4 hours). Assigned reading included publications related to Hospice, selected minutes of meetings of the Board of Directors and the Joint Conference Committee, and the National Cancer Institute proposals (total 5 hours).

To promote familiarity with the rationale and therapeutics employed by Hospice in patient/family care, team members participated in a seminar (total 6 hours) about Hospice goals led by Hospice staff. They also attended lectures on symptom assessment, methods of symptom control, and evaluation of the care plan (total 4 hours). Selected tape recordings of inservice programs were also made available to team members (total 3 hours).

To promote learning and demonstration in an interdisciplinary setting, the program provided for the assignment of each new staff person to each member of the continuing care team, for two days, during which time the new person would be introduced to other staff members and the facilities (total 86 hours). Approximately 32 hours of participation in clinical conferences were also required to meet the objective of interdisciplinary learning.

New members learned about team dynamics through attendance at daily report sessions and clinical conferences (total 30 hours), and a volunteer orientation session (total 4 hours).

To familiarize team members with Hospice policies and procedures, required reading was assigned, including a personnel handbook and policy and procedure manuals (total 2 hours). The individual was assigned to the referral intake unit under the supervision of the Intake Secretary to learn to interpret the criteria for referring sources (average 4 hours). Attendance at three weekly admissions meetings and at a meeting of the Board of Directors was also mandatory (total 5 hours).

To enable the staff member to demonstrate patient/family care skills in the home setting, each new staff person spent two weeks practicing independently, making home visits, being on call, and following up on the plan of care for the currently ill and the bereaved (total 50 hours).

Inservice education sessions were held to familiarize the continuing care team member with health care delivery systems and resources in the local community. The sessions included discussion of agreements and contractual relationships with the Visiting Nurses Association and introductions to the resources and personnel of agencies such as American Cancer Society, Goodwill-Easter Seals, Homemaker Services Bureau, Meals on Wheels, and the Connecticut Mental Health Center. Hospital-based home care programs and the organizational structure of hospitals as they relate to Hospice activities were also studied.

At the conclusion of the six-week orientation program an evaluation was made by the immediate supervisor of both the performance of the new staff person and the effects of the program on the participant.

Content. The program focused on cancer as a major health problem, and the physical and psychosocial effects of the disease and its treatment upon the patient and his family. Emphasis was given to methods of intervention to meet the physical, psychosocial, rehabilative, and spiritual needs of the terminal cancer patient and the family.

The practicum included experience in: (1) identifying the needs of the patient and his family, (2) planning, implementing, and evaluating an approach to patient care, and

(3) coordinating the continuing care efforts of other health care specialists and community resources. Concurrent clinical experiences ensured, as much as is possible, the direct application of the scientific principles learned.

One of the important components of the educational program is the exploration of the health care specialist's attitudes and feelings toward the terminally ill. Health workers must recognize and attempt to deal with personal feelings concerning cancer, pain, loss, and death before they can help the dying patient and the family. Group discussions and individual conferences between the learner and the preceptor explored the learner's feelings about cancer, pain, loss, dying, and the experience of caring for the terminally ill. Such discussions helped the learner recognize and perhaps modify previous attitudes, and enhanced insight into patient and family needs and concerns.

Special Educational Needs. The six-week orientation program was aimed at staff employed at the time the NCI contract was awarded as well as additional staff employed during the first contract year. The program, which was planned with the input of the continuing care team, focused on the educational needs peculiar to the various disciplines and groups represented on the team.

Hospice physicians could regularly attend medical meetings at Yale-New Haven Hospital, including weekly grand rounds and an oncology course (offered every year). These physicians also met weekly with a Yale-New Haven Hospital radiation therapist and other specialists to keep current with advancing knowledge.

In the first 18 months the Hospice social worker's expertise in family assessment, knowledge of psychosocial dynamics in family and group settings, and organizational skills contributed to the identification of the social work needs of the Hospice program. In the second 18 months it was necessary to expand social work. A new social worker was hired who became directly involved with patient/family care. To update and expand her family therapy skills, she attended weekly seminars in the community and met with the Hospice psychiatrist weekly for one hour to review the family caseload.

The orientation program for the secretarial staff is directed at developing the in-house office management necessary for the smooth, day-to-day functioning of the organization. However, part of the orientation period is focused on the clinical area because the secretary acts as the referral intake person, has direct telephone contact with patient/families and professionals in the community, and monitors the whereabouts of the members of the continuing care team in the event of an emergency call.

Orientation for Home Care Staff

The Home Care orientation program is geared to acquaint the staff with their responsibilities and to help them feel secure in the working environment of the program.

The orientation program was designed so that Home Care staff members would become knowledgeable about:
1. the philosophy, objectives, and services of the Home Care program
2. the overall structure of Hospice and the role and functions of the director,

administrator, staff coordinator, and staff in
the Home Care team.
   3. the legal and ethical responsibilities
that pertain to the Home Care program
   4. the agencies commonly used in
coordination of the Hospice Home Care program
   5. the work of each staff person in
Hospice

Continuing Education for Professional Staff

   Supplementing the initial training course,
a bimonthly program of continuing education for
the professional staff was developed to inform
the team of new advances and techniques in
cancer care and care of the dying.
   The program included conferences, seminars,
and workshops; guest lectures; educational
courses sponsored by health care providers at
the local, national, and international levels;
and the Hospice inservice education programs,
which are held on a regular basis. The specific
programs for continuing education in the 1974-77
period are listed below.

Conferences, Workshops, Seminars

Foundation of Thanatology: Two-day seminars on
     various aspects of terminal care.
     November 1974: Nursing Care of the Dying
     Patient in the Home Setting. Seminar
     address delivered by Dorothy Sommers,
     Director of Studies, St. Christopher's
     Hospice, London, England.
     April 1975: The Role of the Social Worker
     in Meeting the Needs of Terminally Ill
     Patient and Family. Seminar included
     lecture on the bereaved child by Edna
     Furman, author of A Child's Parent Dies.

Convocation for Leaders in the Field of Death
     and Dying: Four-day conference to develop
     appropriate standards for care of the
     terminally ill, and explore steps necessary
     to evaluate success. Held at Columbia,
     Maryland, November 1974.
St. Christopher's Annual Conferences: A work
     and training experience at London Hospice,
     held in May.
Hospice's "Day Away" Conference: One day every
     three months set aside for entire staff to
     discuss issues of concern.
Quality of Life Workshop: Dr. Ned C. Cassem,
     Jesuit priest and psychiatrist, discussed
     ethical issues in health care delivery.
     Held at Hospital of St. Raphael, New Haven,
     February 1975.
Second International Convocation for Leaders in
     the Field of Death and Dying: Work was
     undertaken on three documents: Essential
     Characteristics of a Hospice Program of
     Care; Guidelines for Developing a Hospice
     Program; and, Standards of Patient Care
     and Outcome Measures. Held in New Haven.
Symposium on Bereavement: Led by Colin Murray
     Parkes, M.D.; sponsored by Yale School of
     Epidemiology and Public Health and
     Hospice, Inc.
Nursing Seminar on Care of Patients Receiving
     Chemotherapy: Sponsored by Project ONE,
     Waterbury Hospital, Waterbury, Connecticut.
Community Health Services Seminars: Quarterly
     seminars on issues relating to Home Health
     Agencies, sponsored by Association of
     Community Health Service Agencies.
Foundation of Thanatology Conference on
     Volunteer Programs.
First, Second and Third National Hospice
     Symposia: Held in New Haven, Connecticut;
     at Riverside Hospice, Boonton, New Jersey;

39

and Marin Hospice, Kentfield, California.
Work Experience at the Palliative Care Unit,
    Montreal, Canada: Attended by Hospice
    physician for one week.
Palliative Care Conference: three days,
    Montreal, November 1976.
Lecture/Workshop. Day-long program conducted
    by Dr. Elisabeth Kubler-Ross in Boston,
    Massachusetts.
Seminar on the Child and Death: Special
    emphasis on the symptoms and fears of
    terminally ill children and the treatment
    required. Held at Waterbury Hospital.

Guest Lecturers in the Field of Cancer Care and Care of the Dying

Patricia Downey, Rehabilitation Physical
    Therapist, Marie Curie Foundation, England.
Dr. Edward Gilbert, Radiation Therapist,
    Presbyterian Hospital, Denver, Colorado.
Joan Gilbert, Director, Cansurmount Volunteers,
    Denver, Colorado.
Sheila Hanna, Director of Volunteers,
    St. Christopher's Hospice.
Barbara Hill, Executive Director, Hospice of
    Marin.
Dr. Elizabeth Kubler-Ross: Day-long workshop
    focused on stages of the dying process in
    relation to children and adults. Held at
    Hospice. Attendance: 600.
Dr. W. Lamers, Medical Director, Hospice of
    Marin, Kentfield, California.
Richard Lamerton, Medical Director, St. Joseph's
    Hospice, London, England. Discussed long-
    term results of program structuring,
    training methods, and continued development
    of professional relationships.
Eileen MacDonald, R.N., Home Care Team,

Palliative Care Unit, Royal Victoria
Hospital, Montreal, Canada.
Eileen Mann, Matron, St. Luke's Hospice,
Sheffield, England.
Ann McGuigian, R.N., M.S., Public Health Nurse
Consultant, Mental Hygiene, State of
Connecticut Department of Health.
Dr. Balfour Mount, Medical Director, Palliative
Care Unit, Royal Victoria Hospital,
Montreal, Canada.
Colin Murray Parkes, M.D.: Social psychiatrist
and consultant at St. Christopher's
Hospice. Discussed design and objectives
of the bereavement program.
Irene Paulin, R.N., Cansurmount Volunteers,
Denver, Colorado.
Dr. Cicely Saunders, Medical Director,
St. Christopher's Hospice.
Dr. John C. Scott, Palliative Care Unit, Royal
Victoria Hospital, Montreal, Canada.
Consultation with continuing care team
in the clinical field to make observations
and recommendations. April 1975.
Dorothy Sommers, Director of Studies, St.
Christopher's Hospice, London, England.
Discussed the role of the nurse as
coordinator of the total care plan for
patient/family. Spent two days with
Hospice staff.
Reverend Carleton Sweetzer, Chaplain, and
Roberta Paige, both of St. Luke's Hospice,
New York, New York: Discussed problems
and progress in the introduction of Hospice
care within the framework of a large acute-
care hospital. July 1975.
Professor Eric Wilkes, Medical Director,
St. Luke's Hospice, Sheffield, England.

Educational Courses Sponsored by
Health Care Providers

Yale-New Haven Hospital Medication Course for
Senior Licensed Practical Nurses.
Curricula: Metrology, Pharmacology, and
Administration of Medicines; 50 classroom
hours. Taught by the Yale-New Haven
Departments of Inservice Education and
Pharmacy. Attended by Hospice L.P.N.s.

One-Month Course: St. Christopher's Hospice,
London, England. Attended by Home Care
Coordinator, the course provided
opportunities to participate in the total
care of the dying patient and family within
the setting of a Hospice. Program included
two weeks of experience in outpatient
department of St. Joseph's and
St. Christopher's Hospices.

Ten-Day Nurse Attachment Course: St.
Christopher's Hospice, London. Attended
by a Hospice L.P.N. in October 1974, the
clinical experience focused on techniques
of bedside nursing care of the dying
patient within a Hospice setting.

"On Death and Dying": Course conducted by
Elisabeth Kubler-Ross, M.D. Held on a
quarterly basis, the course is a week-long
intensive educational experience on the
awareness and understanding of death.

First International Congress on Patient
Counseling: Variety of workshops including
Dr. Cicely Saunders' program on Death and
Dying. Four-day conference held in
Amsterdam, Holland, in April 1976.

Individual instruction in physical examination
and diagnosis: Dr. David Connell, a
primary care physician, spent one month
with the team giving nurses special

42

instruction on making assessments in the home without the presence of a physician.

Hospice Inservice Education Programs

Dorothy Brubaker, M.S.W., Hospice Social Worker. Topic: "Personality Structure," "Coping Mechanisms," and "Social Class Identification."

Robert Brubaker, M.D. Topic: "Alcoholism"-- detection, community resources, problems.

Robert W. Buckingham, Hospice Research Coordinator. Topic: "Development and Implementation of a Data Base."

George L. Cohn, M.D., Psychiatrist at West Haven Veterans Administration Hospital, Associate Professor of Clinical Psychiatry and Medicine at Yale University School of Medicine. Case Conference: "The Bereaved Adult: How Can We Help Them and When Do They Need Psychiatric Care?"

Dr. James T. Collins, Therapeutic Radiologist, Yale-New Haven Hospital. "Palliative Radiation"--importance of teaching patient/family about therapy, side effects, alterations in physiology, etc.

Sue Cox, Hospice Director of Volunteers. Topic: "Nurse Volunteers"--legal, policy, and procedural considerations of the program.

Judith D'Afflitti, M.S.N. Topic: "Anxiety"-- manifestation in family structures and effects.

Sister Mary Kaye Dunn, Hospice Home Care Coordinator. Topics: "Hospice Patient/ Family Record," "The Problem Oriented Method of Charting," and discussion of forms.

Charlotte Gray, R.N., Hospice Inservice Coordinator. Topic: "Nursing Problems Associated with Care of the Patient with

Head and Neck Cancer," including a film
presentation.

T. Hitchcock. "Interviewing, Part I"- Basic
principles; with C. Collins, "Interviewing,
Part II."

Harold Klein, M.D., Community-based psychiatrist
and consultant at local elementary schools.
Topic: "Bereaved Children: How Do We Help
Them and When Do They Need Psychiatric
Care?"

Sylvia A. Lack, Hospice Medical Director.
Topics: "Pain Control," "Care of the
Patient in Pain."

Dr. Richard Lamerton, Medical Director of St.
Joseph's Hospice, Topic: "Ethics of
Terminal Care."

Arthur G. Lipman, Ph.D., Director of Yale-New
Haven Hospital's Drug Information Center
and Hospice Consultant Clinical Pharmacist.
Sessions on Analgesics, Sedatives and
Hypnotics, Dynamics of Pain, Indications
for Steroid Therapy, Chemotherapeutic
Agents, Antibiotics.

Dr. Colin Murray Parkes, Social Psychiatrist,
Tavistock Institute, London, England.
Case Conference: "Bereavement."

Dennis Rezendes, Hospice Administrator. Topic:
"Third Party Reimbursement."

Sister Margaret Rapson and Sister Jennie Penson,
The MacMillan Unit, Dorset, England.
Program with these visiting British nurses
featured exchange of ideas in areas of
clinical care, reimbursement, organizational
design, and program development.
The MacMillan Unit is a separately funded
palliative care/hospice unit under the
auspices of Christchurch Hospital.

Dr. John C. Scott, Palliative Care Unit, Royal
Victoria Hospital, Montreal, Canada. Topic:
"The Development of a Therapeutic Community."

James Shure. Topic: "Jewish Ritual around
Death and Bereavement"--explanation of
Jewish law and procedures for preparation
of body, services, mourning period,
unveilings.

Ronald Skeel, M.D., Oncologist, Yale-New Haven
Hospital. Topic: "Supportive Medical
Care for the Advanced Cancer Patient."

Anne Smith and Frances Dittes. Topic:
"Creative Movement."--relaxation techniques,
discussion with demonstration and
participation.

Morris A. Wessel, M.D., Pediatrician. Topic:
"The Bereaved Adolescent: Particular
Problems of This Stage of Life and How
We Can Help Them."

Team presentation. "Problem Oriented Medical
Record"--American Hospital Association
requirements, legal aspects, and
components.

CORRECTIONS

On page 267 the second sentence in the last paragraph should read as follows: "Primary care persons were, in general, also more hostile and <u>more</u> anxious and depressed than patients."

Also, under "Acknowledgments" on page xi, the name of Dr. James <u>Jekyl</u> is misspelled.

CHAPTER 5

Volunteer Program,
Director of Volunteers Marjorie Sue Cox

Hospice has demonstrated that volunteers can be an effective, integral part of the interdisciplinary team which cares for terminally ill patients and their families. By supplementing the professional staff's responsibilities and providing services that enhance the care of patients and families, this unpaid segment of the team has become essential to the realization of Hospice goals. Volunteers bring a special gift of self to dying patients and their families. They are caregivers who can honestly say, "I am here because I want to be here."

HISTORY

In April 1974, a Director of Volunteers was hired as part of the original health care team. Marjorie Sue Cox, the director, was chosen on the basis of her own background as a volunteer as well as on her experience as a volunteer director in a health care facility, which gave her the needed insight for selecting applicants of all ages and educational levels and for planning and coordinating the volunteer services.

The director immediately began interviewing volunteer applicants to select a core group to participate in the design and development of the program. Ten volunteers, of diverse ages, backgrounds, and socioeconomic levels, were selected to work closely with the director and other staff to determine how the Hospice program should be organized to enable volunteers to respond effectively to the needs of patients and their families, and to decide what kinds of tasks might appropriately be performed by volunteers. The director also visited St. Christopher's and St. Luke's Hospices in England to observe their volunteer programs.

By the end of the first year, the volunteer program had been developed and met existing legal and health care rules and regulations; 24 volunteers had been trained for direct patient and family care; and an additional 22 volunteers were working in planning, community relations, public reception, research, and on special task forces. The slow and careful development of the program contributed to a solid base for providing services that meet the standards of every discipline, that help to keep down the cost of health care, and that enhance the total care plan.

For the volunteer programs of hospices that are now being planned, a growth similar to that experienced in New Haven would be desirable: namely, that a full-time Director of Volunteers be selected as part of the original staff, that volunteers participate in the planning of the program, that the quality of volunteer services be of the highest priority, that clinical and nonclinical staff be able to work with volunteers, and that the number of volunteers increase slowly.

POLICIES

Legally, the program is an organizational substructure which supplements the paid staff's responsibilities. Volunteers do not replace paid positions; the patient caseload and the planning workload are determined by the available time and expertise of paid personnel. Volunteers provide additional services which enhance the care of families and improve the working environment.

Volunteers are accepted one at a time for the dual purposes of individualized training and integration into the community. Effective teamwork requires that all personnel know each other well. Quality patient care and efficient office management are sustained by team understanding of each individual's strengths and limitations.

All applicants for volunteer service are interviewed by the Director of Volunteers. The only exceptions are special task forces organized by the Board of Directors for specific projects such as fund-raising and inpatient facility planning. The rationale for this policy is to insure that volunteers understand the total Hospice program before beginning service in one department, and that people are placed in jobs that best utilize their skills and individuality. This encourages commitment, job satisfaction, and a sense of effective integration into the Hospice community.

RECRUITMENT AND TRAINING

Most Hospice volunteers apply for service after learning of the program from public speaking engagements and educational programs in the greater New Haven area. Because much of this educational effort is directed toward professional groups, Hospice has attracted health care professionals as well as non-professionals. There is a waiting list of applicants wishing to work directly with patients and families. Thus, active recruitment is necessary only when an unusual skill or talent is required.

As the primary goal is to ensure quality service for patients and families, the numbers of new volunteers must increase slowly so that high levels of communication, thorough training, and continuity of service can be maintained. At this phase of the organization's development the number of volunteers working directly with patients has been limited to a maximum of two per staff person.

The greater New Haven area has a Council for the Directors of Volunteers of all health care and service agencies that use volunteers. The council meets monthly to share programming; this encourages a knowledgeable referral system between agencies and institutions. Occasionally, an applicant has skills, interests, and personality more appropriate for service in another agency and may be directly referred. Through the council volunteer directors can properly place individuals for service and can help ensure that agencies obtain the volunteer expertise needed.

Application Procedure

The Director of Volunteers schedules a two-hour interview with each volunteer applicant. The purposes of the initial interview are to discuss the Hospice history, philosophy, and goals; explain the work of various departments

and the opportunities for volunteers; explore
the background, interests, and skills of the
applicant; learn why the person wants to
volunteer at Hospice; and have the application
form completed.

All applicants are urged to attend the
"First Thursday" orientation to Hospice and are
given selected reading materials about Hospice
including Lack's Philosophy and Organization of
a Hospice Program and Craven and Wald's Hospice
Care for Dying Patients.

Applicants with special skills in
administration, fund-raising, public information,
or research may be referred to the appropriate
department director for an interview, if there
is need for the applicant's skills. If the
applicant is accepted, the department provides
specialized training, supervision, and support.

Applicants who wish to work directly with
patients and families are placed on the waiting
list. As new patient and family needs arise or
as attrition among the volunteer corps occurs,
applicants with appropriate education,
experience, and skills are selected for participation in a group course of several two-hour
sessions conducted by the Director of Volunteers.
The course covers the Hospice program and
philosophy, the volunteer's role in the program,
emotions about death, and procedures in dealing
with patients.

Orientation Course

The orientation course is designed for
qualified applicants who wish to work directly
with patients and families. Six to eight
applicants meet with the Director of Volunteers
for four sessions to learn more about Hospice
care and how they might participate, to explore

their feelings about disease and death, and to discuss listening techniques. The course is a further opportunity for both the applicant and the director to screen the applicant's suitability for direct caregiving before visiting patients' homes with staff. The course protects patients and families from exposure to persons who lack understanding of their problems, protects the caregiving staff from wasting time and energy on unsuitable applicants, and prepares the volunteer for helping people who are experiencing disease, dying, and grief. The fact that, of all the individuals who took the course and still wished to proceed with training for direct patient/family care, only three dropped out during training is proof of the effectiveness of the course as a prescreening tool.

After the course, the Director of Volunteers and the applicant meet for a two-hour interview. The purposes of the meeting are to assess the course, discuss the applicant's suitability for direct patient and family care, agree on the type of assignment, and formally accept the applicant as a home care volunteer. Some applicants decide during the course that they wish to work not as direct caregivers but in tasks that support the program, such as detailed office work. Volunteers are assigned to departments by the Director of Volunteers. Specialized training and supervision is the responsibility of department personnel. Volunteers are invited to participate in inservice education opportunities planned for their department and to become involved in the planning, development, and evaluation of department programming.

Most volunteers who complete the orientation course are found suitable for direct patient and family care. In the postcourse interview the director explains the procedures, policies, and various forms. The volunteer then accompanies experienced caregivers into patients' homes for the training procedure. The volunteer keeps a record during this training--noting the date, the staff person, and the families visited--to enable the director to check the staff person's notes in the patient/family record when questions arise. Staff members evaluate the volunteer trainee's progress and report to the director. This equips the director with essential information for periodic meetings with the trainee.

The training process is complete when the clinical staff and the trainee agree that the volunteer is ready for assignment. Volunteers understand that they will be assigned to a patient or family in need of their particular skills. Some volunteers must wait for months for their first assignment, during which time they continue their reading, attend conferences and inservice education sessions, undertake in-house projects, and attend Hospice social functions.

This thorough method of orientation and training has evolved during the three years of Hospice experience. The training process requires much time, but the result is quality service for patients and families.

CURRICULUM

Session I. Two hours.
Topics:
History of Hospice development
Philosophy, goals, characteristics of a
    Hospice
Categories of Hospice service
Criteria for acceptance into the program
Interdisciplinary staff and volunteer
    expertise
Interagency cooperation
Hospice organization
Assignment of reading list.
    Applicants are required to read the
    following books during the weeks of
    the orientation course: On Death
    and Dying, Questions and Answers on
    Death and Dying, and Death--The Final
    Stage of Growth--all by Elisabeth
    Kubler-Ross, and Bereavement--Studies
    of Grief in Adult Life, by C. M. Parkes.
    Volunteers are encouraged to continue
    reading in the area of their interest
    choosing from books and articles in the
    Hospice Resource Center.

Session II. Two hours.
Topics:
Introductions. Applicants are asked to
    describe their interests, families,
    and why they wish to work with dying
    and grieving persons.
Discussion. Comments and questions from
    the reading list.
Exploration of feelings about disease and
    dying. In every group session the
    following questions have stimulated
    thought and discussion:

54

1. If you could choose when you would
   die, when would it be? When would
   you not want to die? Why?
2. If you could choose how you would
   die, how would it be? How not?
   Why?
3. Thinking of that person with whom
   you are most close, who would you
   want to die first? Why?
4. What do you fear most about dying?

Using a blackboard to write the answers,
   the group will produce a list of all
   the problems associated with the
   entire patient/family caseload.

Using the list, the leader discusses the
   frustration of patients and families
   who are coping with terminal illness--
   the sense of unfinished business,
   unfulfilled dreams, injustice, why me,
   why now, no time for working out the
   meaning or purpose of my life,
   isolation, pain, dependency, loss of
   physical or mental control,
   deterioration, immobility, indignity,
   the wrong person is dying, the one
   whose loss the family can least
   tolerate, financially, emotionally,
   physically, or socially.

Using the list, the leader may point out
   how the expertise of the entire
   interdisciplinary team is needed to
   help patients and families.

Session III. Two hours.
   Topics:
   The gift of self. Caregivers must know
       themselves so that they can be free
       to concentrate on the needs of
       patients and families. A consistently
       useful stimulus has been the

assignment of designing a personal
coat of arms. Applicants are asked
to draw the shape of a shield with
six spaces therein. In each space
they draw a symbol for the answers to
the following questions:
1. What is your greatest strength
   or source of strength?
2. What would the most significant
   other person in your life
   describe as your greatest
   strength or source of strength?
3. Think of three words that
   describe you positively and
   make one symbol.
4. What three words would the
   significant other person use
   to describe you positively?
5. What was your greatest fear as
   a child?
6. What is your greatest fear now?
During discussion the leader points
out the need for caregivers to define
and emphasize their positive traits
and to deal with their fears. To help
patients and families, caregivers must
be sure of their own identities and
recognize their own fears of dying and
grief. This work of developing self-
knowledge must not be done while in
the caregiving role. For this reason
Hospice has developed formal and
informal personal and professional
supports for caregivers, which are
discussed at this session.

Support and communication. The first
support to a volunteer is training by
experienced caregivers for as long as
the applicant desires. This
opportunity provides the individual

with direct exposure to selected
families in the role of observer. It
is a time for identifying strengths
and limitations to determine what type
of assignment would be appropriate for
the individual and therapeutic for the
client. Training takes from two to
five months depending on the individual
and his or her experience with disease,
dying, and grief. This process also
allows staff and volunteer to become
acquainted in preparation for future
personal and professional sharing.
The second mechanism for support is
knowledge. Trained volunteers are
included in clinical conferences,
daily report meetings, and inservice
education sessions. Volunteers are
encouraged to improve their skills and
increase their knowledge in their area
of interest through use of the Hospice
Resource Center and scheduled meetings
with clinical staff. For volunteers
who are unable to attend the weekly
clinical conference, Hospice offers a
monthly evening conference with clinical staff present. Volunteers
assigned to a case have access to the
chart and are kept up to date on the
case by the primary nurse.
Among the informal supports, the clinical
staff is accessible to the volunteers
for discussing questions or problems.
Caregivers are encouraged to share
personal or work-related problems when
they occur with persons in the most
appropriate discipline. Volunteers
also share their problems with one
another.
Volunteers bring to staff the gift of self,

commitment, and caring. Because they
are scheduled for between one and
three days a week, they help in the
refreshment of full-time staff. At
the end of a long, harried day of
patient and family crises a nurse may
turn to a volunteer during a period
of relaxation. Volunteers also
support staff by taking on innumerable
tasks such as filing and Xeroxing.

Session IV. Two hours.
    Confidentiality. The public is keenly
        interested in the details of Hospice
        care. Therefore, personnel working
        with Hospice must be especially
        sensitive to the importance of strict
        patient/family confidentiality.
        Staff and volunteers who work
        directly with patients and their
        families must maintain a rigid silence
        on patient and family information,
        even within their own families.
        Patients and families are discussed
        only with the Home Care Team, and to
        avoid error a list of Home Care staff
        and trained volunteers is given to
        the applicant.
    Active listening. The dying or grieving
        person has the same basic needs as
        anyone else--for life, for safety and
        security, for belonging and affection,
        and for respect and self-respect.
        The caregiver may be called upon to
        respond to these basic needs of the
        patient and family.
    The most important skill for the volunteer
        is to know how to listen to help
        people identify problems and
        communicate where they need help.

An effective caregiver must learn not
only to listen to words, but also to
"listen" to eyes, body language,
family interaction, the environment,
and silence.

Active listening techniques:

1. Show external signs of listening
   by eye contact, nodding appropriately, smiling, gestures, posture.
2. Ask open-ended questions: "I
   don't think I understand" or,
   "What do you mean?"
3. Ask questions that clarify what
   the other person wants to
   communicate, not what you hope
   he is leading up to.
4. Allow time for silence and thought;
   calm silence helps to build trust.
5. Observe signals that a person
   wants to talk: leaning forward,
   seeking eye contact with you,
   pursing their lips; invite them
   to talk.
6. Listen within the framework of
   the other person's purpose;
   seemingly light social conversation may be leading to a concern
   or it may also be a need for a
   light social conversation.
7. As you listen to the words, be
   equally aware of the person's
   nationality, color, religion,
   experience, conditioning, and
   feelings.
8. Use words the speaker uses
   insofar as possible.
9. Especially when the person is
   expressing only incomplete ideas,
   repeat the gist of what he says
   so he can realize how far he's

progressed with the idea and can
continue further if he wants to.
10. If words expressing feelings are
used, form a question such as,
"You said that made you feel
'alone'; what do you mean?"
Allow the person to expand or not,
as he chooses.

Discussion of reading list.

VOLUNTEER ASSIGNMENTS

The need for volunteer service in total
health care is evident in light of the problems
and concerns of patients and families trying to
cope with terminal illness at home. A typical
list of identified problems frequently calls for
the expertise of physician, nurse, social
worker, clinical pharmacist, and clergy, and may
also require the coordination of cooperative
service by many community agencies. There are,
however, areas of clinical and nonclinical concern not covered by existing health care and
service agencies. It is these areas for which
the Hospice volunteer program is designed.

Volunteers are assigned to serve in the
following areas:

Direct Patient/Family Contact
1. Regularly scheduled friendly visits to
help ease the problem of social
isolation and offer a "trained and
empathetic ear"
2. Drop-in visits on evenings and weekends
to check on the condition, desires, and
support of family or friends
3. Escort and transportation assistance
for patients and family members for
necessary appointments and social out-
ings

4. Assistance with homemaking tasks when fatigue or finances are making these a problem
5. Staying with patient or children to allow the primary care person a sleep or social break from patient care
6. Nurse escorts into unsafe neighborhoods or when nursing care requires an aide or when emotional support of the family unit requires two caregivers
7. Bereavement visiting when a relationship has been developed during the illness

On-Call Services

1. Special skills such as home hairdressing or expertise in arts, crafts, or games for remotivation and socialization
2. Area host families willing to provide temporary housing for out-of-town family members of patients
3. Drivers for patient/family errands such as medicine and supplies, food shopping, laundry, and equipment delivery
4. Homemakers to prepare meals and do laundry in their homes for delivery service by other volunteers

Staff Support

1. Typing, filing, mass mailings
2. Hostesses for meetings, seminars, workshops
3. Library and resource center assistance
4. Public receptionists
5. Staff errands
6. Special task committees
7. Babysitting for children of volunteers

Projected Assignments at Inpatient Hospice

1. Indoor and outdoor gardens: planning, planting, maintenance
2. Daily care of patient and public areas to maintain homelike atmosphere: flower arrangements, current magazines
3. Altar Committee: care of candles, eucharistic supplies, hymnals, vestments, programs, bulletins, flowers in chapel
4. Musicians for worship services
5. Cafeteria and gift shop assistants
6. Preparation, decoration, entertainment, and assistance with serving for holiday parties and special events such as picnics, anniversaries
7. Assistants in the day care center for staff and family children
8. Library and resource center workers
9. Patient care: bedside sitting, listening, reading, letter-writing, wheelchair escort around the Hospice and gardens, checkers, chess, cards, etc.
10. Physical care assistants: trained assistants for nurses
11. Hairdressers
12. Entertainers: choral and instrumental musicians, drama groups, dancers
13. Typing and office work
14. Hostesses for meetings, seminars, workshops
15. Pool of area families willing to provide temporary emergency housing for out-of-town family members of patients
16. Holiday tray decorations and tray favors
17. Pool of instructors in arts and crafts.

18. Sewing groups to make patient gowns, lap robes, drapes, and do weekly mending
19. Meal assistants
20. Hospice auxiliary to hold cake sales, craft fairs, and operate coffee bar for public relations and fund-raising for special items needed for patient enjoyment
21. Physiotherapy and occupational therapy
22. Official guides and receptionists
23. Personal laundry care assistants
24. Training and support of new volunteers

Nurse Volunteers

Hospice nurse volunteers offer a wide variety of essential services to patients and families who must cope with terminal illness at home.

Although volunteer nurses cannot use their professional skills without special training to comply with legal and insurance regulations, their contribution lies in their observational skills and previous experience.

Nurse volunteers may drive seriously ill patients to doctor and clinic appointments, sometimes remaining during the examination conference to ask questions and provide moral support. For many patients, the presence of a trained nurse gives reassurance and can help make the difficult waiting room hours tolerable, and even pleasant. The volunteer nurse is also invaluable for sitting with patients. Her expertise provides peace of mind and her presence allows family members an occasional social outing, time alone, or much needed rest.

Registered and licensed practical nurses who want to use their nursing skills as volunteers must complete an additional

specialized training process to ensure that
their performance meets the standards set for
Hospice staff nurses. The training includes
15 hours of seminar conducted by the clinical
staff, after which the nurses travel with staff
members for evaluation in three levels of
professional skills.

Bereavement Program

Until the spring of 1977, bereavement
follow-up was done by the Hospice Home Care
staff. It had become apparent, however, that
this task could be done more economically and
with equal effectiveness by a group of specially
trained volunteers. Since that time a program
for the training of bereavement volunteers has
been instituted and is now an integral part of
volunteer activities.

Selection Criteria. The original nine-
member Hospice Bereavement Team was selected
using the following criteria:
1. They were trained Home Care volunteers
    and thus understood the procedures,
    policies, and philosophy of Hospice
    Home Care, and they knew the clinical
    staff who cared for the patients and
    their families during the illness.
    (All Home Care volunteers have gone
    through a six-week training/selection
    process.)
2. They had maturity, sensitivity, appro-
    priate motivation, and were not in the
    first year of bereavement themselves
    due to a major personal loss through
    death, divorce, etc.
3. They were likely to remain in this area
    for a number of years. The team will
    be used for the training of additional

bereavement volunteers as the need increases.
4. They were of diverse backgrounds: male, female, all ages, various occupations.
5. They committed themselves to attendance at six initial training sessions and ongoing bimonthly education/support meetings.

Training. The training of the team included six two-hour lectures by the Hospice staff: The Medical Director, psychiatrist, social worker, nurse, volunteer clinical psychologist, volunteer community pediatrician, and two bereaved persons. The curriculum covered normal grief, atypical grief, morbidity, mortality, special situations such as loss of child, loss of parent, loss through suicide, death and the child, death and the adolescent, family response to loss, family interactions.

Procedures. The program is coordinated by one of the volunteer team members, who is responsible for record keeping, scheduling, and the assignment of volunteers. After the death of a patient, the staff nurse schedules one or two visits to the bereaved person(s). The nurse determines the need for referral to the Bereavement Team for follow-up. The coordinator matches the appropriate volunteer to the case based on the volunteer's available time and the assessed number of visits per month which will be needed.

The clinical consultants to the Bereavement Team are the Hospice Medical Director and psychiatrist who meet with the group or with individual members as needed, usually at least once per month. Day-to-day support and super-vision are provided by a volunteer clinical psychologist who is available one day per week

in person or at any time by phone. The team
meets bimonthly as a group for team development,
inservice education, and discussion of cases.
These meetings are co-chaired by the volunteer
coordinator and the volunteer psychologist.

Upon assignment to a new case, the
volunteer reads through the patient/family
record and then schedules an interview with the
primary nurse if there are specific questions
or unusual problems which need clarification.
Visits to the home are scheduled by phone or
mail. The frequency of visits is determined by
the bereaved person's needs and the range is
usually once per week to once per month. The
follow-up may occasionally be accomplished by
telephone calls only.

Hospice Bereavement Team members are not
therapists. They have been trained to recognize the normal grieving process and to offer
support by actively listening while the process
is worked through. They also recognize
symptoms of atypical grief and, in consultation
with the Hospice clinicians, can make referrals
for appropriate professional assistance. The
therapeutic value of knowing someone understands
and accepts the feelings and behavior of normal
grief and will continue regular contact through
the acute bereavement period is often all that
is needed for a healthy return to one's own
lifestyle.

Team responsibilities are often in areas
of resocialization and remotivation. During
the acute period of grief, the volunteer often
accompanies the bereaved person through the
maze of legal, insurance, and financial affairs
which must be settled. During this time, the
volunteer will begin to try to learn what the
lifestyle and interests of the person were
before the illness and death of the loved one.
With sensitivity to the person's right to

determine the pace of return to the old
lifestyle, the volunteer encourages
resocialization and often accompanies the
bereaved person to community resources such
as senior centers, social clubs, religious
services, volunteer or employment placement
centers, adult education opportunities.

In this manner, Hospice follows the
survivors of patients through the acute period
of grief. The follow-up support may be as
short as one month or longer than one year.
Discharge planning is determined in consultation at team meetings and usually includes a
phase-out period of less frequent visits or
replacing visits with an occasional telephone
call. Eventually the client is asked if
discharge is agreeable. People are always
discharged with the invitation to call if
problems occur; in that event, the case is
reopened. The team initiates contact with
discharged persons by telephone or note at
three months, six months, and just before the
one-year anniversary of the death.

Exhibit C

STATISTICAL SERVICE PROFILE
September 1, 1976 - June 1, 1977

Total number volunteers during nine months	71
Average roster of volunteers available	
for service each month	55
Net total recorded service hours	7,100

Direct Patient/Family Care:

Total number trained for direct care	32
Average roster of volunteers available	
for service each month	24
In training	9
Total number patient/family units served	52
Total number visits*	650
Total number recorded hours of service**	1,477

Volunteer Corps Profile

Female	59
Male	12
Median age	46.7
(Oldest age 80, youngest age 22)	
Education:	
Doctoral level	3
Master's level	3
Bachelor's level	30
Two years technical training	
or college	25
Employment:	
Registered nurse	17
Licensed practical nurse	2
Full-time employed	17
Full-time students	5

* Does not include evaluation interviews or staff escorting

** Does not include travel, charting, reporting, conferences

THE HOSPICE VOLUNTEER AND
THE PATIENT/FAMILY RECORD

Policy:
There must be a written entry into the
Patient/Family Record of every volunteer service
provided for Hospice patients and families.
It is the responsibility of clinical staff
to read and countersign a written entry into the
Patient/Family Record made by a volunteer.

Procedure:
1. Who may have access to the Patient/
    Family Record? Only the specially
    trained Home Care Volunteers may have
    access to the Patient/Family Record.
2. Who may chart on the Patient/Family
    Record? All specially trained Home
    Care Volunteers are to enter their
    notations directly onto the Patient/
    Family Record.
    Other volunteers who provide services
    to Hospice patients are to report the
    service(s) performed to Hospice staff
    who will then enter a notation of the
    service(s) in the Patient/Family
    Record, e.g. errands, equipment
    delivery, meal preparation, etc.
3. Format. The format of notations made by
    volunteers is to comply with Hospice
    policies and procedures as detailed in
    Section One of this manual.
4. What are the methods of entering the
    volunteer's written notation into the
    Patient/Family Record?
    a. Direct Entry. A volunteer is
        encouraged to return to the Hospice
        Office after a visit to enter
        notation(s) in the Patient/Family

69

Record whenever feasible based on economy of time and travel and Hospice office hours.

b. Indirect/Delayed Entry. Exceptions to (a) are in those instances in which: the visit(s) is made outside of regular office hours; or the location of the visit results in an uneconomical expenditure of time and travel for the volunteer to return to the Hospice office to enter notations in the Patient/Family Record.

IN WHICH CASE:

a. Telephone Report:

No Significant Change. If the volunteer's visit is one which in his judgment there are no significant changes based on the "pre-visit" report by staff to the volunteer, the volunteer need not telephone report until the next regular office hour.

This report is then entered into the Patient/Family Record by a member of the Home Care Staff, with the detailed written report to follow by the volunteer.

Significant Change. If, in the judgment of a volunteer based on a "pre-visit" report from staff, the volunteer assesses a "significant change" in the patient/family condition, the volunteer shall use discretion as to whether to phone Hospice Clinical staff immediately in

70

the course of the visit, or
immediately thereafter.

The report of the volunteer's
assessment that a significant
change has occurred shall be
entered into the Patient/Family
Record by the clinical staff,
with the volunteer's written
report to follow for entry into
the Record.

b. Delayed Written Entry:

In the case of exceptions to a
the volunteer's written report
is to be hand-delivered or mailed
to the Hospice Office as soon as
possible.

Exhibit E
STATEMENT OF POLICY ON INSURANCE COVERAGE
FOR VOLUNTEERS

Professional Liability:

The Hospice insurance package includes the work of trained volunteers registered with the Director of Volunteers.

1. The professional services which may be provided by a volunteer will be limited to specific areas of expertise and skills defined by the Hospice staff.
2. A volunteer working directly with patients and families will complete an extensive training program, will have defined limits of activity, and will work under the direction and supervision of Hospice staff.
3. Hospice insurance covers only that defined service within the limits set for each individual volunteer.
4. The volunteer will be personally responsible for any activity beyond the specific directions given by staff.
5. Volunteers whose professional discipline requires licensing or registration must have on file at Hospice a copy of their current license or registration before rendering professional services to patients and families.

Personal Liability:

Hospice carries a blanket liability policy for registered, trained volunteers. The limits for personal injury or property damage liability, or both combined, are $1,000,000 for each occurrence. The total annual limit is $3,000,000.

Accident Insurance:

1. Hospice recommends that volunteers carry personal health and accident insurance.
2. When a volunteer is injured while performing services for or at Hospice, she or he is legally entitled to limited medical coverage from the agency.
   a. Hospice does not provide workmen's compensation insurance for volunteers.
   b. Hospice does provide accident insurance coverage for volunteers up to $2,500 per volunteer.
   c. If injury is caused by negligence, the individual whose negligence caused the volunteer's injury is personally liable, and the volunteer can recover from the person whether or not the person is an employee of Hospice.

Automobile Liability:

1. All volunteers who use their automobile for Hospice business must have $100,000/$300,000 personal liability coverage on the automobile.
2. Applicants must provide a copy of their automobile insurance policy for their personal file before acceptance as a Hospice volunteer.

CHAPTER 6

Procedures

Several types of services are available within the Hospice program including the Full Scope patient care program, Pain or Medical Consult, Nursing Consult, and Relative Consult.

To be eligible for the Full Scope service patients must meet the following guidelines:

1. The diagnosis must be terminal cancer
2. The prognosis must be six months or less
3. The patient must live within the service area
4. The primary doctor must give consent and cooperation
5. The patient and family must give consent
6. Preferably there should be a primary care person, although this is not mandatory

Exceptions to these criteria can be made if Hospice services are appropriate to meet a particular family's needs.

Referrals come from varied sources ranging from the primary doctor, Visiting Nurse Association, hospital nurses, social workers, other agencies, family members, and occasionally from the patient.

Patient/Family Admission

The Admissions Registrar takes all incoming referrals. Calls are screened and cases not meeting guidelines can be directed to appropriate resources within the community. Families outside the Full Scope service area may be eligible for Medical, Nursing, or Relative Consult services. When all criteria have been met the referral is placed into the cleared category in order of need.

Those patients and families whose needs are most urgent are assessed as soon as possible. Each Tuesday at Patient Care Conference, remaining referrals are reviewed for the staff and assignments are made for assessments for the following week.

Following this the R.N. or L.P.N. visits the patient and family and assesses their eligibility. If they are to be accepted a history and physical are obtained, and notes are made concerning the patient's needs, such as diet and activity, and family needs. A medical release form is signed. The nurse then explains the team concept, including on-call availability, and leaves the names of the team members and a phone number to call if necessary before the next visit is made.

A chart is then made up and a record number assigned. Patient and family needs are listed in numerical order so that they can easily be

referred to or added to. Medications and any-
thing else requiring a physician's orders are
charted to await verification. The Hospice
Admissions Order Form is mailed to the primary
doctor for his signature. This lists patient
and family needs noted by the nurse, medications
and other orders, and a care plan. Upon it's
return, this form is checked and signed off by
the R.N. shift coordinator. On the same or the
next day the referral source (if not the patient
or family) and the primary doctor are telephoned
to notify them of the acceptance in the Hospice
program. The Visiting Nurse Association, if
indicated, and any other pertinent agencies are
also called and a provisional care plan is
prepared.

That day at the daily report the staff on
duty are given a brief report on the new case.
If necessary, immediate visits are scheduled at
this time.

At the next Tuesday Patient Care Conference
the case is presented to the entire interdisciplinary team including R.N.s, L.P.N.s,
doctors, a social worker, and the volunteer
director. The case is assigned to a primary
care nurse according to case load. The team
discusses plans and reviews whether the social
worker or physical therapist is needed, after
contact and verification of the primary doctor,
and how volunteers may be used. At the Tuesday
Conference the team also handles the discharge
of cases.

The primary nurse becomes responsible for
future contacts with doctors and other agencies,
keeping the chart in order and updated,
recording order changes, and sending a Hospice
Progress Report sheet to the primary doctor
every six weeks or sooner if necessary to keep
him aware of the patient's condition and to
renew orders. In the absence of the primary

nurse, the nurse in charge that shift becomes
responsible for any changes. Accordingly the
R.N. or L.P.N. working the shift is responsible
for contacting the next R.N. shift coordinator
about changes in orders in the condition of the
patient.

After the death of a patient, a visit is
made to the family as soon as possible and
always within one week. At that time the
primary care person is scored using Dr. Colin
Murray Parkes's Questionnaire which identifies
families who are likely to undergo problematic
bereavement. If the primary care person scores
above 18 on this instrument, they are assigned
to a specially trained member of the volunteer
bereavement team. Often, when a primary care
person is thought to be a potential high risk
an attempt is made to introduce this volunteer
even prior to the death so that a rapport can
be established.

Procedure Manuals

In the course of establishing the program
of services, many procedures had to be developed
and approved. Three manuals incorporating
policies and procedures for all aspects of
Hospice care have either been developed or are
now being completed. These manuals will provide
Hospice staff with the necessary tools to
deliver and evaluate the program services.

The Hospice Patient/Family Record Policies
and Procedure Manual. The manual explains in
detail the policies and procedures for the use
of the Patient/Family Record. The record is a
modification of the Problem Oriented Medical
Record System developed by Lawrence Weed, M.D.,
University of Vermont.

In its treatment of the policies governing

78

the use of the record, the manual emphasizes
the legal and accepted standards of practice for
use of medical records. The record manual has
been approved by the Medical Advisory Committee
and is evaluated and reviewed annually by the
Clinical Policy Review Committee.

Because of the legal and confidential
nature of patient records, the policies governing their administration, method of entry,
accessibility, and use are explicit. An excerpt
from the manual's Record Policies on the
following pages will illustrate its content.

The second section of the record policies
and procedure manual contains detailed
instructions for the use of each form in the
record. An example of such instructions is
shown in the exhibit on the following pages,
an excerpt from the manual's Care Plan
instructions.

The Hospice Chemotherapy Manual. The
chemotherapy manual was developed by Hospice
staff nurses and has been approved by the
Hospice Medical Advisory Committee. It serves
as a quick and easy reference for clinical staff
for their own information and for the education
of patients and families. This manual will be
reviewed semi-annually and amended as necessary
to aid staff in their awareness of current
changes and trends in chemotherapy. The manual
also provides a place to log suggestions based
on experience in the administration of chemotherapeutic agents in the home setting.

The manual includes statements on Hospice's
philosophy in regard to chemotherapeutic agents,
significant points regarding the education of
patients and their families about these drugs,
how to answer some of the most frequently asked
questions about the palliative/therapeutic
aspects of these drugs when administered in

terminal phases of cancer and Hospice policies in regard to these agents, and other issues related to appropriate care for the dying.

The second part of the manual contains profile sheets on the most commonly prescribed chemotherapeutic agents in Hospice's experience to date. Each sheet contains information regarding indications for use; nature, route, strength, and dosage; side effects; and special nursing and teaching points on administering an agent. Staff are encouraged to record on these profile sheets any significant findings or help-ful hints in their experience with the agent.

The Hospice Clinical Policies and Procedure Manual. This manual is the largest and most comprehensive of those developed to date. It contains the composite of the medical, nursing, social service, volunteer, pastoral care, home health aide, speech, occupational, and physical therapy, and administrative policies and pro-cedures related to the day-to-day operation of the Home Care Program. This manual should be considered to be standard and is similar to the standard operational manual of any Certified Home Health Care Agency such as that of a Visiting Nurse Association.

EXCERPT FROM HOSPICE PATIENT/FAMILY
RECORD POLICIES AND PROCEDURES MANUAL

Record Policies

1. All Hospice staff, consultants, volunteers, and/or persons providing service under contract are required to enter notations in the HP/FR regarding services provided.

2. If an entry cannot be made into the HP/FR immediately following the provision of the service, a telephone call shall be made by the provider to the Shift Coordinator or her designated representative with a written report to follow as soon as possible.

3. All services offered but refused are to be recorded as such. For example: "Bed bath offered but refused by patient." ...

4. The HP/FR is a legal and confidential document. Only authorized Hospice personnel and selected trained Home Care volunteers may have access to the HP/FR.

5. It is the responsibility of clinical staff to read and countersign a written entry into the HP/FR made by a volunteer.

6. The HP/FR as a legal document is the only written evidence that care was or was not provided. From a legal standpoint, if care to the patient/family is not recorded, it is contestable that the care was provided.

7. All telephone calls relative to the delivery or coordination of service to a patient/family are to be recorded in the HP/FR.

8. There must be written physician orders available in the chart for all services requiring written orders.

9. It is illegal to erase a written entry in the HP/FR. Errors should be circled with "error" written above the circle thusly:

> "Mr. Jones said he did (not) want to try once again to learn how to give the medication to his wife."

EXCERPT FROM HOSPICE PATIENT/FAMILY
RECORD POLICIES AND PROCEDURES MANUAL

Care Plan

The Care Plan is the specific intervention designed to meet the needs of the patient/family.

The Care Plan is physician-directed and under the clinical supervision of the Patient Care Coordinator or her designated representative.

The Care Plan is identified by the primary nurse in consultation with other professional disciplines represented on the Hospice team and the Director of Volunteers in situations where the services of a volunteer are desired.

The Care Plan should be <u>clear</u> so that there is no question in the minds of members of the team as to what is to be done.

The Care Plan should also be <u>specific</u> to the need it is intended to meet.

Finally, the Care Plan should be <u>inclusive</u> of the skilled and specialized care being provided by a Hospice program.

The Care Plan is reviewed as often as necessary with a minimum of once a week at Clinical Conference for patients who are currently ill and a minimum of once every four weeks for the bereaved.

When a particular treatment or procedure has been found to be effective when done a certain way, the description of the technique is written in the Care Plan so that all Hospice nurses can be familiar with it and the patient can have the benefit of a consistent approach to the performance of the treatment or procedure.

Each Care Plan that is designed to meet a particular patient/family need (see List of Needs) is assigned to the same number as the need. For example: number 3 on the List of Needs should have intervention to meet that need numbered 3 on the Care Plan as well. There must be a Care Plan for each identified need and, in many cases, there will be more than one Care Plan to meet a need.

Illustration:

Need #3: To prevent sacral decubiti from external irritation.

Care Plan

#3 Teach patient and family various positions of comfort so that patient can tolerate being on sides and abdomen for longer periods of time.

#3 Teach primary care person the method and importance of keeping sacral area clean and dry.

#3 Teach primary care person the proper technique of massaging the area peripheral to decubiti. NEVER RUB THE REDDENED AREA!

General Instructions:

1. The number of the need for which the intervention is designed is written in the column on the left of page.

2. The date the intervention was incorporated into the care plan is written in the column to the right of the date.

3. The initials of the nurse or other clerical personnel making the entry in the chart are written in the signature column to the right of the date.

4. The Care Plan is written in the space to the right of the signature.
5. When a Care Plan is discontinued, i.e., the need is resolved, a red line is drawn through the Care Plan with the date the need was met and the initials of the person discontinuing the Care Plan written in Red Ink at the end of the red line.

CHAPTER 7

Summary: Essential Features of Hospice Services

Hospice, Inc., New Haven, and the National Cancer Institute (NCI) have demonstrated that home care is very much desired by a proportion of the population. There was concern at the outset of the program that palliative home care would be unacceptable in this country. Hospice planners were frequently told that Americans are hospital oriented, that "when Americans are sick they want to be in the hospital. Nobody dies at home in this country; the society isn't set up for it." Yet Hospice personnel have found that families are prepared to accept great hardship to keep a loved one home; that (at the appropriate time) intensive personal care or palliative care is welcomed by patients and their families; and that a service emphasizing the quality of life rather than diagnosis and cure can be accepted and integrated into

professional and lay concepts of health care.
Moreover, the evaluation study has shown that
this service benefits patients and families
alike and that the benefits are measurable.
This achievement has not come easily; many
mistakes were made along the way. Grappling
with innovative changes caused inevitable
inefficiencies in the use of staff time.
Through its contract with the NCI, however,
Hospice was able to develop, free from the
usual financial and bureaucratic constraints, a
program that does, in fact, meet the needs of
patients and their families.

CHARACTERISTICS OF A HOSPICE PROGRAM OF CARE

Certain program characteristics have
evolved from the experience of the last three
years. These, listed below, are essential to
the delivery of effective Hospice care to the
terminally ill and their families:

1. Coordinated home care, with inpatient
    beds under a central autonomous Hospice
    administration

2. Control of symptoms (physical, socio-
    logical, psychological, and spiritual)

3. Physician-directed services

4. Provision of care by an inter-
    disciplinary team

5. Services available on a 24-hour-a-day,
    7-day-a-week basis with emphasis on
    availability of medical and nursing
    skills

6. Patient and family regarded as the unit of care

7. Bereavement follow-up

8. Use of volunteers as an integral part of the interdisciplinary team

9. Structured personnel support and communication systems

10. Patients accepted to the program on the basis of health needs, not ability to pay

Home Care--Inpatient Facilities

The New Haven Hospice began life in a very different fashion from any then-existing hospice. For three years home care was provided without any back-up beds. This was a non-threatening method of introducing the concept to the health care community, as few of them operate in the home at all. The participation of Visiting Nurse Associations in planning the program and their willingness to share the care in many homes was crucial to providing optimal terminal care. Among the benefits of VNA involvement was that it permitted an expansion of the notions of what is possible in home care. During the study period more than 65 percent of patients died at home--much above the national average. Yet despite the radical departure from the usual locale of care, there was never any controversy with established medical opinion about the appropriateness of such deaths. Hospice experience also bore out the original contention that terminally ill patients require care of an intensity not usually provided by nursing homes. Of the 34 percent who did not die at home, only three percent died in nursing homes.

Disadvantages were many. Many patients adamantly refused to go into a facility, usually because on previous admissions they had experienced a deficiency in the type of intensive personal care they needed. Several of these died at home with symptoms that could have been controlled in a hospice facility. Other home deaths created a very great strain for the family. In addition, there was symptomatic deterioration of many patients following hospital admission. Continuity of care was lost and techniques of comfort that worked well in the home were ignored by a system geared to investigation, diagnosis, and care--but not to comfort care. The past three years' experience indicates that optimum hospice care can be delivered only when home care and inpatient beds are under the same central, autonomous hospice administration.

On the North American continent there have been several innovative approaches to providing these two components. Hospice is following the St. Christopher's model of building a 44-bed hospital to provide a therapeutic environment uniquely qualified to back up the Home Care Program. At the Royal Victoria Hospital in Montreal, Dr. Balfour Mount has created a 14-bed Palliative Care Unit within an acute-care general hospital. The unit functions largely as a separate entity, with its own philosophy of care and the relaxation of many hospital regulations. St. Luke's Hospital in New York City has taken yet another approach. It provides an interdisciplinary hospice team which attends the terminal patients in the hospital wherever they may be located. Special provisions are made for hospice patients in terms of family and children's visiting, hairwashing, and the like.

The team works closely with the ward staff to provide the best care for the patient and follows the patient and family in the home setting.

Symptom Control

Among health care professionals and those concerned with the issues of death and dying there is far too much talk about psychological and emotional problems of dying patients, and far too little about the physical comfort of these patients. Any group concerned with service to the dying should be talking about smoothing sheets, rubbing bottoms, relieving constipation, and sitting up at night. Counseling a person who is lying in a wet bed is ludicrous. Discomfort looms large in the lives of patients with a terminal illness and must be of importance to physicians and other health care providers if they are to treat the whole person.

If people are cared for with common sense and basic professional skills, with detailed attention to self-evident problems and physical needs, patients and families can themselves cope with many of their emotional crises. Without pain, well-nursed, with bowels controlled, mouth clean, and a caring friend available, the patient will be able to bring the psychological problems into manageable perspective.

Any physician who is dealing with a number of terminally ill patients must become concerned with symptom control and skilled in the management of the various types of physical distress caused by an incurable illness. Sadly, the terminal stage has been defined by some as beginning at the moment when the doctor says, "There is nothing more to be done," and then begins to withdraw from the patient. Patients,

of course, are well aware of when this happens.
There is never a time when "nothing more can be
done." There may indeed be nothing more that
can be done to cure the disease, but there are
always further measures to be taken for the
comfort of the patient and the well-being of the
family.

Severe cancer pain can be controlled by
narcotics and adjuvant drugs. The narcotic
should be titrated to the patient's need and
used regularly to maintain pain control. Taken
in regular oral doses, a narcotic can be used
for many months without a need to escalate the
dose. Hospice has demonstrated that regular
narcotic use is accepted by doctors and patients
and that oral morphine is a good substitute for
oral heroin. (In May 1977, St. Christopher's in
London changed from oral heroin to oral morphine.)

Every physician dealing with these patients
should have a virtually inexhaustible store of
remedies for all the common problems of terminal
disease. A problem-oriented approach is useful--
treating each symptom almost as a disease in
itself to be diagnosed and treated. Thus the
patient is not Mr. A., with incurable cancer, but
Mr. A., the man with the severe pain for which a
great deal can be done. This enables the team
to approach the patient with a positive,
optimistic, realistic attitude. The benefits
from such an approach for the patient and family
are often dramatic.

Physician-Directed Services

It is vital to the psychological and
physical well-being of the patient with terminal
illness that the physician be a key figure
throughout the care program. Patients with a
terminal illness and their families consistently
report their feelings of abandonment by medical

personnel. A new Hospice patient said sadly, "Well, I feel as though I have lost Dr. Q. somewhere along the way." There is a time in a patient's illness when the health care professionals begin to feel that there is nothing more that they can do, and it is the loss of their doctor's interest that patients fear the most. If a patient elects to remain at home for his last weeks, this decision frequently cuts him off from effective medical care because many physicians do not make home visits. Many seriously ill patients, suffering from vomiting, pain, and other controllable symptoms, bedfast at home, have not seen a doctor for many weeks. Others find that if they do struggle to the office or to a hospital clinic, they are frequently seen by a resident while the person they regard as their doctor is seeing patients who can be cured.

Medical direction of the Hospice program was also vital in gaining acceptance by the medical community. Fears were expressed by physicians at the start that, once referred to the Hospice program, patients would be on a "one-way escalator to death" regardless of improvements in their condition or new advances in treatment. To the contrary, Hospice, New Haven, demonstrated that competent medical overview identified misdiagnoses, remissions, complications amenable to hospital treatment, and patients referred too early in the course of their disease.

Provision of Care by an Interdisciplinary Team

The care of the dying must be a team concern. The team includes the dying patient, his or her immediate family, the doctor, the chaplain, the nurses, the social worker, the volunteers, and other health care personnel.

Continuity of management forms an important part of the total care. Interdisciplinary care must not be synonymous with fragmented care, in which the bewildered patient does not know who is dealing with which problem. Real teamwork mandates that the interdisciplinary staff have regular conferences to work out a plan of care for patients and families and to learn one another's professional languages.

Teamwork depends upon the support and supply staff, without whom the frontliners would collapse. On the first Hospice home visit, personnel explain the team concept and prepare a handwritten list of the team personnel, which is to be placed by the phone. Recently, on reading the list, a wife exclaimed, "But what about Kay and Jill [Hospice secretaries]? They are the only ones who've helped me so far." Hospice personnel have learned that it is only by constant listening to the patients and family members that they can even approach an understanding of the basic components of good care.

Hospice seeks to complement, not duplicate, the services tendered by others. There is no room in terminal care for interagency rivalries or interdisciplinary turf guards. Attitudes of openness and cooperation and the philosophy of an extended team help to maintain good working relationships with other essential agencies and personnel. Two examples of the extended team in New Haven are the Visiting Nurse Associations and the community pharmacists (one of whom made Dilaudid suppositories from cocoa butter on a weekend after 17 phone calls had failed to locate any). Imaginative individuals prepared to go to extraordinary lengths for a person in pain help make Hospice work.

Service Availability on a 24-Hour Basis

The experience of the families regarding
available help must tally with what they are
told. "You're very difficult to get hold of,"
insisted one daughter. She was trying in vain
to tell her mother's physician that, prior to
the present admission, she had tried to reach
him for three days because her mother had
severe vaginal bleeding. Finally, a dash to
the Emergency Room resulted in immediate
admission. No amount of reassurance by the
doctor, as he tried to persuade her to take
mother home again, could blot out the fear and
anxiety of those three days. Families
occasionally test out Hospice's 24-hour
availability and call for help at an unusual
hour for some trivial reason. Once they dis-
cover that Hospice personnel really are there,
they stop testing and do not abuse the service.

Patient and Family Regarded as the Unit of Care

Objective support for this concept now
comes from the evaluation study, which indicates
that the family member primarily carrying the
burden of care suffers more anxiety, depression,
and social malfunctioning than the patients
themselves. This was true in both Hospice and
non-Hospice groups. (see Part III, Findings.)
"Nothing that we do should serve to separate
someone who is dying from his family," Dr.
Cicely Saunders, St. Christopher's director, has
said. "There may be moments of difficulty or
even despair, but it is of paramount importance
that they come through to the end together. The
journey itself may ease the next stages for
those who have to go on living afterwards."
A terminal illness is not like an acute illness.

In an acute illness, although the short-term stress may be great, the long-term hope and anticipation is that full family function will be restored and life will go on as it did before. In a terminal illness every member of the family is pulled in and affected by the illness. Adjustments to living without the patient begin before death, as functions previously fulfilled by the patient have to be taken over by other members of the family. Thus the family should be involved from the beginning.

On the patient's admission to an inpatient facility, family members who have been nursing the patient at home have invaluable experience and advice to offer the professionals on the precise details of care: which is the most comfortable position, how frequently medication needs to be given to keep pain under control, certain expressions unique to this particular patient. For example, a 19-year-old was labeled confused and was heavily sedated after he had repeatedly cried out in a terrified fashion that a big red engine was in the room. It was only after his death that the family mentioned that the fire service had brought his oxygen to the home when he had had breathing difficulties. He was trying to communicate to the hospital staff a need for oxygen and help in breathing. He was not asking to be sedated.

Many family members deny their own needs because of the demands of looking after the sick person. Their own needs still exist, however, and they worry about them. Eventually they feel neglected and may resent the patient for drawing attention away from themselves. Time spent listening sympathetically to a patient's husband telling of his fears for his own health because he has been passing blood in his urine for two months is time well spent.

Over and over again Hospice staff hear

families say, "We could not have done it without
you." One woman said that the Hospice staff
were her "backbone." "You held me up so that my
hands were free to care for my father," she
said. Families can manage for a much longer
period of time if they have professional
support immediately available to them.

Bereavement Follow-up

Care does not stop with the death of the
patient. A Hospice program provides emotional
support for families during bereavement.
Through the National Cancer Institute contract
Hospice, New Haven, was able to test the need
for this element of the program in this country.
Through trial and error, Hospice developed a
unique program combining early follow-up by the
primary nurse and long-term follow-up by
volunteers. The family is visited on a scheduled or emergency basis through the death and
on into the mourning period. Unfortunately,
time and funding did not permit bereavement
follow-up to be included in the evaluation
study, but this is the next area that should be
evaluated.

Bereavement follow-up is preventive health
care. Families require assistance as they
endure the suffering caused by the separation.
In the first year after bereavement there is
increased vulnerability to illness, reflected in
a 40 percent increase in the mortality rate of
widowers. Other consequences include increased
alcoholism, reactive depression, and long-term
detrimental effects to children caused by loss
of a parent. Dr. Colin Murray Parkes believes
that simple friendly visits that give the
survivors an opportunity to express their grief
and discuss the terminal illness and death can
go a long way toward mitigating the ill effects

of bereavement.

In this program the first bereavement visits are made by the primary nurse who cared for the patient before death. The nurse's presence gives the family an opportunity to discuss questions such as, "Should we have kept him at home? Should we have taken him to the hospital? Was it worth continuing with that unpleasant treatment for so long? Should we have pressed him to continue with chemotherapy? Why didn't she go to the doctor as soon as she felt the lump?" Many of these questions can easily be cleared up by frank and open discussion. Left unattended they grow and fester in the minds of the bereaved to cause much unnecessary suffering. Subsequent visits are made by trained volunteers.

Volunteers: An Integral Part of the Home Care Team

"You medical folk are all very nice," said one husband, "but the real people are better." Lay volunteers can help the family with the day-to-day tasks of running a household, with housework, shopping, or babysitting. They can help with laundry, patient transportation to outpatient clinics, and many other apparently small, but essential, jobs--the tasks that the family member is pulled away from by the demands of caring for the patient.

The volunteer is also uniquely able to help the patient maintain or reestablish his sense of self-worth. Dependency, the lack of independent functioning created by a disability, eats away at a person's self-esteem. The withdrawal of health care professionals as they try to cope with their own feelings of inadequacy reinforces the patient's diminishing sense of worth. The volunteer, by forming a close, friendly relationship, can counteract this process.

Hospice, New Haven, gives volunteers a basic orientation to the program but does not attempt to have them function as counselors for the dying. Their special value is as a person with whom the patient can identify. The patient sees them as "people like myself." Patients discuss many topics with the lay volunteers which they would not discuss with the professionals, either because they feel these concerns are too silly to bother the doctor with or that the doctor has no time to attend to these concerns or would not understand them. For one of Hospice's patients, doctors, nurses, social workers, and psychiatric services had all been employed in an attempt to help him and his family deal with their many problems. All efforts were consistently rejected. The only person who was accepted and helpful was the volunteer who took the patient fishing and in the course of those trips discussed, on a person-to-person basis, the philosophies and fears the patient was encountering.

Structured Personnel Support and Communication Systems

If personnel are to form close human relationships (the foundations of hospice work), they must experience a kind of support not usually found in health care agencies. But within this general framework there are many unanswered questions: How should Hospice select staff? Why do people come to work at Hospice? Why do they stay? Why do they leave? Hospice, New Haven, has developed some functional approaches to staff support, based on its three years' experience. Quality inservice education, the team approach, administration-clinical communication, regular conferences--formal and informal--an occasional "day away" for all staff, an active volunteer corps, part-timers, and the monitoring of workloads to prevent burnout syndrome among overzealous staff--these are a few of the mechanisms used for staff support.

Patients Accepted on Basis of Need

Patients are accepted on the basis of health care needs, not on ability to pay. No British hospice discriminates against patients because of their financial status, and American hospices must also strive to uphold this high standard of care. American hospices cannot avoid responsibility in this area by any reference to socialized medicine: Most of the hospices in Britain are not under the National Health Service. Rather, they are financed by a combination of donations, patient contributions, and government reimbursement.

One example of the financial dilemma facing patients with terminal illness is illustrated by the problem of a Hospice patient who died this year, a 38-year-old, first-generation Italian immigrant, a husband and father of three children. The patient was paying off $12,000 in hospital bills at $50 a month. He owned his own home. Like many Hospice patients, he was too young for Medicare and too rich for Medicaid. He could have disposed of his assets to become eligible for Medicaid, but he and his wife were counting on their small family business and home to provide for the needs of their family after his death.

There is a gaping void in our health care delivery system. Hospice and the National Cancer Institute have pioneered in developing a program that fills this void, ushering in a new kind of health care. This care has been accepted by the consumer and has been shown

by objective study to improve the quality of
life of patients with a terminal illness and
their families.

PART II

Hospice Patients and Families: A Statistical Portrait

CHAPTER 8

Patient, Family, and Program Characteristics

INTRODUCTION

During the period from September 1975 to June 1977, 170 patient/families received full-scope services from Hospice. "Full-scope" services means that the full interdisciplinary home visiting team described elsewhere in this report was available on a 24-hour, seven-day-a-week, on-call emergency basis. Regular scheduled visits were also made.

The information obtained from the persons in this 170-unit sample provides significant insights into the characteristics of patients and primary care persons, and the types of services provided to them.

Data were collected by Hospice home care personnel who sometimes found it difficult to ask for certain kinds of personal information

from patients or their families. In some
instances, therefore, the totals do not add to
the study population of 170 persons; neverthe-
less, the missing data do not detract from the
overall quality of the information.

CHARACTERISTICS OF PATIENTS
AND PRIMARY CARE PERSONS

Socioeconomic and Demographic Attributes

Patient age. At admission the mean age of
Hospice patients was 64 years. Patients ranged
in age from 30 to 98 years. As table 1 shows,
persons between ages 60 and 64 constituted the
greatest proportion--one-fifth--of all
patients, followed by persons aged 65 to 69,
who represented 19 percent of the total.
        Almost three-fourths of all patients were
in the age group of 55 to 79. Half of Hospice
patients were under 65. This finding has
serious ramifications for future third-party
reimbursements as persons under 65 do not
qualify for Medicare unless disabled for two
years. Few patients in terminal care qualify
under this provision.

Patient sex. Of the 170 patients in the
study population, 56 percent were female and
44 percent were male.

Patient marital status. As shown on
table 2, about two-thirds of patients were
married, and about one-fourth were widowed.

Number of persons in household. Two-
thirds of the patients came from households
where there were either two or three people

(table 3); almost half came from two-member households. Thus the burden of care is borne by the one "healthy" household member although in many cases this person was also in poor, or only fair, health; occasionally that person was also terminally ill. This high percentage of two-member households suggests that the availability of Hospice help eases the burden for the sole care giver.

However, 48 percent came from three- to five-member households where, presumably, more persons were available to help. In some cases larger families need more family aid to sort out disturbed or unhelpful family dynamics.

The mean number of persons in the household was 3.1.

Ethnic background and race. Table 4 shows that 35 percent of Hospice patients are of Italian descent. Almost 16 percent had Irish heritage. Racially, 93.5 percent of patients were white and 6.5 percent were nonwhite.

The proportions of various ethnic groups shown in table 4 are similar to the ethnic mix of the area covered by Hospice

Socioeconomic status. The Hollingshead Two-factor Index (occupation and education) was used to categorize the socioeconomic status of Hospice patients (see table 5). On the Hollingshead scale the numeral I represents the highest social class (in terms of occupation and education) and V represents the lowest. Clearly the patients served during the study period were not in the higher socioeconomic status levels: 90 percent were found in levels III, IV, and V, compared to only 10 percent in classes I and II. Among Hospice patients the dominant social class was IV (45.6 percent), followed by V (29.6 percent).

Particularly significant for third-party reimbursement is the high figure for class IV. These persons usually have poor private insurance coverage and few personal financial resources; yet they do not qualify for welfare and Title 19. Three-fourths of patient/families come from classes IV and V, classes usually requiring above-average social service aid.

Education. Table 6 shows that about one-third of the patients were high school graduates compared to 22 percent who had at least some college, were college graduates, or had advanced graduate or professional training; 45.4 percent had not graduated from high school.

Religion of patient. Table 7 indicates that two-thirds of patients were Catholic, about one-fourth were Protestant, almost 7 percent were Jewish, and 3 percent reported other denominations or had no religion.

This table gave important information to Hospice about the type of pastoral-care person most needed by Hospice families. A Roman Catholic priest has recently been added to the team. The high proportion of Catholics is doubtless due to the large Italian and Irish population in the New Haven area. Other Hospices may need clergy of another denomination or faith.

Length of time since patient last worked. As shown in table 8, about 22 percent of the patients had stopped working within the past six months; 15 percent within the past year. Two patients were currently working. Many had not worked for numerous years: 12 percent had not worked within the past five years and

11 percent had not worked for 10 years. It is assumed that the 17.6 percent who reported that they had "never worked" were, for the most part, housewives.

Primary payment source. Table 9 shows the variety of sources patients used to meet their medical costs. By and large, the greatest proportion of patients used some combination of sources, which consisted of federal aid, voluntary health insurance, and their own personal resources.

About 27 percent relied solely on federal government sources compared to 31 percent who relied only on voluntary health insurance.

Patient residence. Almost a third of the patients resided in New Haven (table 10). More than half were from towns contiguous to New Haven, contributing to increased travel time from the Hospice office in New Haven. The information about the distribution of Hospice families as depicted by this table allowed Hospice administration to assign each nurse a geographical area to cut travel time and increase efficiency. Such an arrangement might be relevant for other Hospices dependent upon their geographical distribution.

Primary care person. The mean age of primary care persons (PCPs) for the patients in the study population was 55.5 years. Table 11 shows that 10 percent of PCPs were under age 30, 15 percent were between ages 30 and 44, and 44 percent were between ages 45 and 64. Almost one-third were 65 or older.

Particularly interesting were the three primary care persons under 20 years old and the five over 80 years. One might not expect to

TABLE 1

Age of Patients

Age	Number	Percentage
All ages	168	100.0
30-34	3	1.8
35-39	3	1.8
40-44	5	3.0
45-49	9	5.4
50-54	10	5.9
55-59	20	11.9
60-64	35	20.8
65-69	32	19.0
70-74	20	11.9
75-79	17	10.1
80-84	8	4.8
85-89	4	2.4
90 and over	2	1.2

Note: Percentages do not total 100% due to rounding.

TABLE 2

Marital Status
of Patients

Marital Status	Number	Percentage
Total	170	100.0
Single	11	6.5
Married	106	62.4
Divorced	7	4.1
Widowed	41	24.1
Separated	5	2.9

TABLE 3

Number of Persons in
Households of Patients

Number of persons in household	Number	Percentage
Total	170	100.0
One	4	2.4
Two	80	47.1
Three	35	20.6
Four	15	8.8
Five	22	12.9
Six or more	14	8.2

TABLE 4

Ethnic Backgrounds
of Patients

Ethnic Background	Number	Percentage
Total	153	100.0
Italian	54	35.3
Polish	11	7.2
Irish	24	15.7
English	11	7.2
Scandinavian	11	7.2
Afro-American	10	6.5
Other	32	20.9

TABLE 5

Socioeconomic Status of Patients

Socioeconomic status	Number	Percentage
Total	125	100.0
I	3	2.4
II	10	8.0
III	18	14.4
IV	57	45.6
V	37	29.6

NOTE: Based on Hollingshead Two-Factor Index of Occupation and Education. On the Hollingshead scale the numeral I represents the highest social class (in terms of occupation and education) and V represents the lowest.

TABLE 6

Education of Patients

Education	Number	Percentage
Total	152	100.0
Graduate or pro-fessional training	1	0.6
College or University graduate	15	9.9
Partial college	17	11.2
High School graduate	50	32.9
Partial High School	17	11.2
Completed 7-9 grades	38	25.0
Less than 7 years	14	9.2

TABLE 7

Religion of Patients

Religion	Number	Percentage
All Religions	165	100.0
Protestant	38	23.0
Catholic	111	67.3
Jewish	11	6.7
Other or no religion	5	3.0

TABLE 8

When Patient
Last Worked

When last worked	Number	Percentage
Total	137	100.0
Working now	2	1.4
Within previous 6 months	30	21.9
One year ago	20	14.6
Two years ago	17	12.4
Five years ago	17	12.4
Ten years ago	15	10.9
Over 10 years ago	12	8.8
Never worked	24	17.6

TABLE 9

Primary Payment Source
for Medical Costs

Primary Source of Payment	Number	Percentage
All sources	162	100.0
Voluntary health insurance	50	30.9
Federal government[1]	44	27.2
Private (personal) resources	2	1.2
Combination[2]	63	38.9
Other or no source	3	1.8

NOTES:
1. Medicare, Medicaid, or Veterans Administration
2. Primarily federal government, voluntary health insurance, and private (personal) resources

TABLE 10

Residence of Patients

Residence	Number	Percentage
All residences	170	100.0
New Haven	52	30.6
East Haven	20	11.8
West Haven	27	15.9
North Haven	8	4.7
Branford	9	5.3
Hamden	29	17.0
Milford	15	8.8
Orange	7	4.1
Woodbridge	3	1.8

TABLE 11

Age of Primary Care Person

Age of Primary Care Person	Number	Percentage
All ages	138	100.0
Less than 20	3	2.2
20-24	4	2.9
25-29	7	5.1
30-34	5	3.6
35-39	6	4.3
40-44	10	7.2
45-49	8	5.8
50-54	3	2.2
55-59	20	14.4
60-64	30	21.7
65-69	17	12.3
70-74	12	9.4
75-79	8	5.8
80 and over	5	3.6

NOTE: Percentages do not total 100.0% due to rounding.

TABLE 12

Relationship of Primary
Care Person to Patient

Relationship	Number	Percentage
Total	168	100.0
Spouse	99	58.9
Child	38	22.6
Sibling	12	7.1
Extended family	10	5.9
Parent	6	3.6
Friend	1	0.6
No primary care person	2	1.2

NOTE: Percentages do not total 100.0% due
to rounding.

TABLE 13

Health Status of
Primary Care Person

Health status of PCP	Number	Percentage
Total	154	100.0
Good	103	66.9
Fair	41	26.6
Poor	10	6.5

find an individual in these age groups bearing the main brunt of terminal care.

The relationship between the PCP and the patient is shown in table 12. The majority of patients were taken care of by their spouses; in 23 percent of the study population the PCP was the patient's child. Brothers or sisters were the PCPs in 7 percent of the cases, and extended family arrangements were stated for about 6 percent of the patients.

Two-thirds of the primary care persons reported their health to be good; one-fourth reported it to be fair; and 6.5 percent said they were in poor health (table 13). It is remarkable that one-third of the primary care givers were not themselves in good health. Practical aid as well as advice and counseling is a necessity in such homes.

Families also indicated that there were other supportive people. The extended family was reported by 69 percent of the study population. Thus, despite its oft-lamented disappearance, the extended family is frequently an important contributor to the care of a person with a terminal illness at home. Five percent of the patients were aided by friends and another five percent by employed help.

Patient Clinical Attributes

<u>Primary disease site</u>. Patients with cancer of the lung, breast, or colon constitute almost half of all the patients in the study population (table 14).

The distribution of primary disease site reflects the common cancers against which disease-specific therapy is relatively ineffective for metastatic disease. Hospice rarely sees varieties of neoplastic disease

for which chemotherapy has become increasingly
important in the past two decades, such as
advanced Hodgkins, choriocarcinoma, acute
lymphocytic leukemia, testicular carcinoma,
and histiocytic lymphoma. Such patients are
cared for by acute oncology centers such as Yale.

Metastatic site. Table 15 shows that in
19 percent of the patients, the metastatic site
was recorded as "bone" compared to 18 percent
"liver," 15 percent in "one or more locations,"
11 percent "lung," and 11 percent "disseminated."
Common cancers seen by Hospice--breast, lung,
and prostate--also commonly metastasize to bone.

Patient status upon admission. About 47
percent of the patients were classified as
ambulatory patients when admitted to the
Hospice Home Care program, compared to 40 percent
who were bedridden and 14 percent who were
ambulatory with some assistance (table 16).
These figures are important. A higher
proportion of bedridden patients would probably
have increased the amount of care required.
It is vital for a new Hospice to educate their
referral sources and to avoid being swamped with
large numbers of acutely ill bedridden patients
referred far too late in their illness. Such
was the experience of several British Hospices,
successfully avoided in New Haven by good
community and professional education.
Almost three-fourths of the study
population were aware of their diagnosis,
compared to 9 percent who were unaware. For
17 percent of the study population, it is
uncertain whether the patient knew of the
diagnosis.
Patient complaints upon admission. Upon
admission, patients were asked about a variety

121

TABLE 14

Primary Disease Site

Primary disease site	Number	Percentage
All sites	170	100.0
Lung	31	18.2
Breast	29	17.1
Colon	23	13.5
Prostate	11	6.5
Pancreas	8	4.7
Kidney	7	4.1
Esophagus	5	2.9
Liver	4	2.3
Ovary	4	2.3
Mouth/Tongue	4	2.3
Stomach	3	1.8
Basiloid - Anus	3	1.8
Larynx	3	1.8
Cervix	3	1.8
Thyroid	3	1.8
Other*	29	17.1

*Includes five patients for whom primary disease site was not recorded; two patients each for: bladder, spine, throat or pharynx, bile duct or gall bladder, Hodgkins disease (lymphosarcoma), lymphoma, lymphocytic lymphosarcoma, jaw or neck, and breast with combination of another site. In addition there were individual patients with the following disease sites: endometrium, glioblastoma (brain), vagina myeloma, abdomen, plus one patient without cancer.

TABLE 15

Metastatic Site

Metastatic site	Number	Percentage
Total	138	100.0
Bone	26	18.8
Liver	25	18.1
Combination	21	15.2
Lung	15	10.9
Disseminated	15	10.9
Brain	7	5.1
Other	18	13.0
Site not stated	15	8.0

TABLE 16

Status upon Admission

Patient status upon admission	Number	Percentage
Total	162	100.0
Ambulatory	76	46.9
Ambulatory with assistance	22	13.6
Bedridden	64	39.5

of conditions. Nine of ten patients reported having diarrhea and drowsiness, edema (88 percent), frequent urination or incontinence (86 percent), and anxiety (86 percent). Eight out of ten patients reported coughing (83 percent), insomnia (82 percent) and nausea or vomiting (79 percent). Three-fourths of the patients cited worry (75 percent) and breath-lessness (74 percent). Constipation was reported by 68 percent, anorexia by 65 percent, weakness by 45 percent, and pain by 33 percent.

UTILIZATION OF SERVICES

Number of Months in Program

Table 17 shows the length of time patients received Hospice services: 41 percent had a "length of stay" in the Home Care program of less than one month, 25 percent received service from one to two months, 18 percent from two to four months, and 15 percent were Hospice Home Care patients for more than four months.

The mean number of days in the program was 70.5, and the range was from one to 630 days.

These figures indicate a satisfactory referral pattern and attest to the efficiency of the screening process. The long-stay patients were mainly those who outlived their original prognosis because of good symptom control, who were referred by Hospice referral for further disease-specific treatment, or who experienced unexpected remission. These patients were kept in the program to provide a stable baseline population.

Number of Visits and Number of Visit Hours

Table 18 indicates that 40 percent of all

patients received less than ten visits compared to 28 percent who received between 10 and 19; 15 percent between 20 and 29; and 16 percent 30 or more visits.

Half the patients received fewer than 10 hours of service from Hospice Home Care personnel (table 19). Almost one-fourth received between 10 and 19 hours; 12 percent, between 20 and 29 hours; and 13 percent, 30 or more hours of Home Care visits and concomitant services.

The correlation between total visits and visit hours is 0.95. The mean number of visit hours was 16.4; the range was 1.0 to 82.4. It would be interesting to study those families who need 30 or more visits to ascertain what family needs elicited more visits from the Home Care team and to evaluate the appropriateness of the greater number of visits.

Type of Visit

Hospice Home Care personnel provide numerous services during their visits to their patients. The types of services that are provided by Home Care personnel during their visits are categorized below:

      Assessment or evaluation visit
      Physical care visit
      Teaching visit
      Social service visit
      Pastoral visit
      Death pronouncement visit
      Bereavement visit
      Discharge visit

During the study period, information was recorded for patients who received bereavement, evaluation, physical care, and social service visits. As shown in table 20, over one-third

125

of the patients' families received four or more
bereavement visits, and one-fifth received
three visits.

Of the 163 patients receiving evaluation
visits, more than half had one evaluation visit;
one-fourth had between 10 and 19 visits (see
table 20).

Physical care visits were made to 150
patients in the sample. Almost three-fourths
received fewer than 10 visits. One-fifth
received between 10 and 19 visits and 8 percent
received 20 or more.

Of the 150 patients who obtained social
service visits, two-thirds received fewer than
10 visits.

To summarize, the mean number of total
visits was 17.8, the median was 12, and the
range was from 0 to 81 visits. For evaluation
visits, the mean number was 12.9, the median
was 8, and the range was from 1 to 71 visits.
The mean number of physical care visits was 8.2,
the median was 5.0, and the range was from 1 to
71 visits. There was an average of 3.8
bereavement visits, the median was 3.0, and the
range was from 1 to 17 visits.

Some comments on these figures are relevant.
The patient with a terminal illness is not in a
stable condition. Advancing disease causes
daily or at least weekly changes in the
patient's physical and psychological conditions.
These changes need constant monitoring and
treatment adjustments to keep the patient
comfortable. Hence the need for repeated
"evaluation" visits. The large number of
physical care visits contrasts sharply with the
British experience. In Britain the district
nursing service does all physical care and the
Hospice nurses give only supportive advice and
counseling. In New Haven, Connecticut, the
Visiting Nurse Association provides physical

care from 8:00 a.m. to 4:00 p.m., Monday through Friday. Thus the Hospice staff must provide physical care nights and weekends.

Many of the social services rendered the patients were done by nurses and might be more appropriately performed by a social worker or aide. Finally, if the family is regarded as the unit of care, the final service provided to the family must be bereavement follow-up.

Place of Death

Table 21 shows the patient's place of death during the study period. Almost two-thirds died at home, compared to 27 percent who died in acute-care hospitals, 3 percent in nursing homes, and 3 percent elsewhere (for example, in an ambulance or boarding home). The number of Hospice patients dying at home rather than in hospitals steadily increased throughout the contract period, standing at over 70 percent in the last three months. This is far above national figures and clearly indicates that patients and their families can undergo a home death if the proper assistance is provided. Of patients not dying at home, most died in hospitals and not in nursing homes --an essential fact to bear in mind when future cost-effectiveness studies are done. The cost of Hospice care must be compared to that of the acute-care hospital and not that of a nursing home.

TABLE 17

Length of Time
in Program

Length of time in program	Number	Percentage
Total	156	100.0
Less than 1 month	64	41.0
30-60 days	40	25.6
61-120 days	28	18.0
121 or more days	24	15.4

TABLE 18

Number of Visits
to Patients

Total number of visits	Number	Percentage
All services	166	100.0
Less than 10	67	40.4
10 - 19	47	28.3
20 - 29	25	15.1
30 or more	27	16.2

TABLE 19

Number of
Visit Hours

Number of hours	Number	Percentage
Total	165	100.0
Less than 10	83	50.3
10 - 19	40	24.3
20 - 29	20	12.1
30 or more	22	13.3

TABLE 20

Number and Types
of Visits

Number and type of visit	Number	Percentage
Bereavement - All	87	100.0
One visit	17	19.5
Two visits	21	24.1
Three visits	17	19.5
Four or more visits	32	36.8
Evaluation - All	163	100.0
Less than 10 visits	86	52.8
10-19 visits	43	26.4
20-29 visits	17	10.4
30 or more visits	17	10.4
Physical care - All	150	100.0
Less than 10 visits	110	73.3
10-19 visits	28	18.7
20 or more visits	12	8.0
Social service	150	100.0
Less than 10 visits	99	66.0
10-19 visits	26	17.3
20-29	13	8.7
30 or more visits	12	8.0

NOTE: Percentages do not total 100.0% due to rounding.

TABLE 21

Place of Death

Place of Death	Number	Percentage
All places	149	100.0
Patient's home	98	65.8
Acute hospital	41	27.5
Nursing home	5	3.4
Other	5	3.4

NOTE: Percentages do not total 100.0% due to rounding.

ASSOCIATIONS BETWEEN FINDINGS

Primary Disease Site

Table 22 shows the relationship between primary disease site and patient age upon admission to Hospice (p = 0.04). Persons in their sixties accounted for the greatest proportion of patients regardless of the primary disease sites (except for breast cancer).

The relationship between primary disease site and the patient's status upon admission to Hospice is shown in table 23; no statistical significance was found. Of patients with lung cancer, 57 percent were ambulatory, one-third were bedridden, and 10 percent were ambulatory with assistance or their status was unknown. Of patients with cancer of the colon 47 percent were ambulatory and 47 percent were bedridden. Breast cancer patients were slightly more apt to be ambulatory than bedridden.

No statistically significant relationship was found between pain and the primary disease site. As table 24 shows, about one-third of lung cancer patients reported having no pain as did 43 percent of those with cancer of the colon, 31 percent with breast cancer, and 28 percent of patients with cancer of other sites.

The relationship between the number of months as a Hospice patient and the primary disease site is shown in table 25. Breast cancer patients appear to have a longer stay on the program than other patients.

Table 26 shows the relationship between primary disease site and total visit hours.

Regardless of disease site, about two-thirds of all Hospice patients received less than 20 visit hours from Hospice personnel. As indicated in relation to table 19, the mean number of visit hours was 16.4. The mean number of visits for all patients was 17.8. Breast cancer patients and patients with cancer of other sites had more visits than did patients with lung or colon cancer. This appears to be a function of their greater length of stay in contrast to patients with lung or colon cancer. It is possible that breast cancer patients are referred to Hospice at an earlier stage because, as breast cancer strikes the homemaker in the family, help in the home is needed sooner.

Table 27 shows the visits of personnel in relation to primary disease site; no statistically significant relationship was identified.

Tables 28 and 29 show the associations between physical care and social service visits and primary disease sites. Breast cancer patients needed fewer physical care visits and more social service visits than did other patients. It may be that a great deal of emotional support and counseling given to breast cancer patients was classified as social service.

The relationship between primary disease site and place of death is shown in table 30. Fewer lung cancer patients died at home than did patients with colon or breast cancer. Shortness of breath, a common symptom in lung cancer, may have precipitated inpatient admissions. Dyspnea is a particularly frightening symptom and very difficult to control at home.

Place of Death

Tables 31 to 38 show relationships between place of death and various patient attributes

TABLE 22

Age of Patient by Primary Disease Site

Age	Total		Primary Disease Site			
			Lung	Colon	Breast	Other
Total Number	(162)		(31)	(23)	(28)	(80)
Total Percentage	99.9		100.0	100.0	100.0	100.1
	%	#	%	%	%	%
30–50	11.7	(19)	19.4	4.4	17.9	8.8
51–60	19.1	(31)	25.8	13.0	35.7	12.5
61–70	38.9	(63)	38.7	43.5	32.1	40.0
71–80	22.2	(36)	16.1	21.7	10.7	28.8
80 and over	8.0	(13)	--	17.4	3.6	10.0

NOTES:

Percentages may not total 100.0% due to rounding.

This table excludes those people (4.7% of total) for whom there was no information regarding either age or primary site.

TABLE 23

Status at Admission by Primary Disease Site

Status at Admission	Total		Primary Disease Site			
			Lung	Colon	Breast	Other
Total Number*	(162)		(30)	(21)	(28)	(77)
Total Percentage	100.0		100.0	100.0	100.0	100.1
	%	#	%	%	%	%
Ambulatory	46.9	(76)	56.7	47.6	42.9	46.8
Bedridden	39.5	(64)	33.3	47.6	35.7	37.7
Other	13.6	(22)	10.0	4.8	21.4	15.6

NOTES:

Percentages may not total 100.0% due to rounding.

This table excludes those persons (4.7% of total) for whom no status at admission was recorded.

*Six persons included in the total had no primary site: five were ambulatory and one was bedridden.

135

TABLE 24

Incidence of Pain by Primary Disease Site

Incidence of Pain	Total		Primary Disease Site			
			Lung	Colon	Breast	Other
Total Number*	(170)		(31)	(23)	(29)	(81)
Total Percentage	100.0		100.0	100.0	100.0	100.0
	%	#	%	%	%	%
No pain	33.5	(57)	32.3	43.5	31.0	28.4
Pain	66.5	(113)	67.7	56.5	69.0	71.6

*Six persons included in the total had no primary site: five had incidence of pain.

136

TABLE 25

Length of Stay by Primary Disease Site

Length of Stay in Months	Total		Primary Disease Site			
			Lung	Colon	Breast	Other
Total Number	(170)		(31)	(23)	(29)	(81)
Total Percentage	100.0		100.0	100.0	100.0	100.0
	%	#	%	%	%	%
Less than 2 wks.	8.2	(14)	3.2	3.2	10.3	8.6
1/2 to 1 mo.	37.6	(64)	41.9	43.5	20.7	38.3
1 to 2 mos.	23.4	(40)	25.8	21.8	24.1	24.7
2 to 4 mos.	12.4	(21)	12.9	13.1	10.3	13.6
Over 4 mos.	18.2	(31)	16.1	17.4	34.5	14.8

NOTE:

*Six persons included in the total had no primary site: all were in the program less than one month.

137

TABLE 26

Total Visit Hours per Patient by Primary Disease Site

Total Visit Hours	Total			Primary Disease Site				
			Lung	Colon	Breast	Other
		#				
Total Number*	(170)		(31)	(23)	(29)	(81)
Total Percentage	99.9		100.0	99.9	99.9	100.1
	%		%	%	%	%
None	2.9	(5)	--	--	3.5	2.5
1 to 9	48.8	(83)	45.2	47.8	51.7	49.4
10 to 19	23.5	(40)	35.5	26.1	17.2	21.0
20-29	11.8	(20)	16.1	13.0	10.3	11.1
30 or more	12.9	(22)	3.2	13.0	17.2	16.1

NOTE:

Percentages may not total 100.0% due to rounding.

*Six persons included in the total had no primary site: four had between 1 and 19 visit hours, two had none.

138

TABLE 27

Total Number of Visits per Patient by Primary Disease Site

Total Visits	Total			Primary Disease Site			
				Lung	Colon	Breast	Other
Total Number*	(166)			(31)	(23)	(28)	(80)
Total Percentage	100.0			100.1	100.0	99.9	100.1
	%	#		%	%	%	%
1 to 9	40.4	(67)		38.7	34.8	46.4	38.8
10 to 19	28.3	(47)		32.3	34.8	21.4	27.5
20 to 29	15.1	(25)		22.6	21.7	10.7	12.5
30 or more	16.3	(27)		6.5	8.7	21.4	21.3

NOTES:

Percentages may not total 100.0% due to rounding.

The table excludes those persons (2.4%) who received no visits.

*Four persons included in the total had no primary disease site: three received between 10-19 visits.

139

TABLE 28

Number of Physical Care Visits by Primary Disease Site

Physical Care Visits	Total			Primary Disease Site			
			Lung	Colon	Breast	Other	
Total Number*	(170)		(31)	(23)	(29)	(81)	
Total Percentage	100.1		100.0	100.0	100.0	100.1	
	%	#	%	%	%	%	
None	11.8	(20)	12.9	8.7	10.3	9.9	
1 to 9	64.7	(110)	71.0	65.2	72.4	60.5	
10 to 19	16.5	(28)	16.1	21.7	13.8	17.3	
20 or more	7.1	(12)	--	4.4	3.5	12.4	

NOTES:

Percentages may not total 100.0% due to rounding.

*Six persons included in the total had no primary disease site: three received no physical care visits; three received between 1-9 physical care visits.

140

TABLE 29

Number of Social Service Visits by Primary Disease Site

Social Service Visits	Total				Primary Disease Site			
			Lung	Colon	Breast	Other		
Total Number*	(170)		(31)	(23)	(29)	(81)		
Total Percentage	100.1		100.0	100.0	99.9	100.0		
	%	#	%	%	%	%		
None	11.8	(20)	3.2	--	27.6	11.1		
1 to 9	58.2	(99)	64.5	69.6	34.5	60.5		
10 to 19	15.3	(26)	25.8	21.7	17.2	9.9		
20 to 29	7.7	(13)	6.5	--	10.3	9.9		
30 or more	7.1	(12)	--	8.7	10.3	8.6		

NOTES:

Percentages may not total 100.0% due to rounding.

*Six persons included in the total had no primary disease site: two persons received no social service visits; four persons received between 1-9 visits.

141

TABLE 30

Place of Death by Primary Disease Site

| Place of Death | Total | | | Primary Disease Site | | | |
			Lung	Colon	Breast	Other
Total Number	(149)		(30)	(22)	(21)	(72)
Total Percentage	100.0		100.0	100.0	100.0	100.0
	%	#	%	%	%	%
Home	65.8	(98)	53.3	72.7	61.9	69.4
Other	34.2	(51)	46.7	27.3	38.1	30.6

NOTES:

This table excludes those persons (12.35%) for whom there was no information regarding place of death.

Four persons included in the total had no primary disease site: three died at home.

142

and characteristics. As shown in table 31, 70 percent of all male patients died in their home as did 62 percent of the females.

No statistically significant relationship was found between place of death and marital status (table 32).

Table 33 shows that, regardless of social class (Hollingshead classification), proportionately more persons died at home than elsewhere: Patients in class V are, however, more likely than others not to die at home.

Table 34 shows the relationship between place of death and the patients' status upon admission to Hospice. Of those who died at home, 40 percent were ambulatory upon admission to the Hospice Home Care program, 43 percent were bedridden, and 17 percent had other status upon admission (usually ambulatory with assistance).

Table 35 relates place of death and number of months as a Hospice patient (length of stay). Of those patients who died at home, 44 percent were in the program for less than one month, one-fourth for one to two months, and 12 percent for two to four months; a somewhat similar distribution is found for patients who died at locations other than their homes. It seems that a longer stay on the program goes along with a home death. This may reflect the longer influence of Hospice in facilitating such an event.

The relationship between total number of visits and place of death is shown in table 36. Of those who died at home, 35 percent had fewer than 10 visits from Hospice personnel, whereas of those who died in locations other than their homes, a much higher percentage (51 percent) had fewer than 10 visits from Hospice personnel. A low percentage of those who died in locations other than their homes had 30 or more visits

143

in contrast to those who died at home, 16 percent of whom had 30 or more visits. It seems that a home death requires more visit hours, possibly because more help is needed to deal with a very sick person at home.

No statistically significant relationship was found between visit hours of Hospice personnel and place of death (table 37).

Table 38 in this series shows the relationship between place of death and the health of the primary care person (PCP). It would be interesting to explore what factors enable a care-giver in poor health to keep a dying relative home until the end. Were there other care-givers in the household, or did Hospice or the VNA increase their coverage?

No statistically significant relationships were found between place of death and race, sources of payment, relationship of primary care person, and age of PCP (tables not shown).

Total Visits

Tables 39 to 42 show the relationships between the number of total visits made by Hospice personnel and selected attributes and characteristics of patient and primary care person (PCP). The mean number of visits was 17.8, the standard deviation was 17.7, and the range was from 0 to 81 total visits.

Table 39 shows the relationship between total visits and sex of the patient. Among men, 36 percent had 20 or more visits, whereas 26 percent of females had more than 20 visits. Possibly more men had lung cancer and needed more visits to attempt to control dyspnea.

An equal distribution of number of visits was found through all social classes (table 40).

A statistically significant relation ($p = 0.0003$) was found in the relationship

TABLE 31

Place of Death
by Sex

| Place of Death | Total | | Sex | |
			Male	Female
Total Number	(149)		(67)	(82)
Total Percentage	100.0		100.0	100.0
	%	#	%	%
Home	65.8	(98)	70.1	62.2
Other	34.2	(51)	29.9	37.8

NOTE: The table excludes those persons (12.6% of total) for whom there was no recorded place of death.

TABLE 32

Place of Death
by Marital Status

| Place of Death | Total | | Marital Status | |
			Never Married	Ever Married
Total Number	(149)		(10)	(139)
Total Percentage	100.0		100.0	100.0
	%	#	%	%
Home	65.8	(98)	60.0	66.2
Other	34.2	(51)	40.0	33.8

NOTE: This table excludes those persons (12.6% of total) for whom there was no recorded place of death.

TABLE 33

Place of Death by Socioeconomic Status

Place of Death	Total	Hollingshead Classification				
		I	II	III	IV	V
Total Number	(112)	(3)	(10)	(15)	(48)	(36)
Total Percentage	100.0	100.0	100.0	100.0	100.0	100.0
	% #	%	%	%	%	%
Home	67.0 (75)	100.0	70.0	73.3	70.8	55.6
Other	33.0 (37)	--	30.0	26.7	29.2	44.4

NOTES:

On the Hollingshead scale the numeral I represents the highest social class (in terms of occupation and education) and V represents the lowest.

This table excludes those persons (34.1% of total) for whom there was no recorded place of death or who were not categorized on the Hollingshead scale.

147

TABLE 34

Place of Death by Status at Admission

| Place of Death | Total | | Status at Admission | | |
			Ambulatory	Bedridden	Other
Total Number	(141)		(62)	(58)	(21)
Total Percentage	100.0		100.0	100.0	100.0
	%	#	%	%	%
Home	66.0	(93)	59.7	69.0	76.2
Other	34.0	(48)	40.3	31.0	23.8

NOTE: This table excludes those persons (17.1% of total) for whom there was no answer on the question regarding status at admission.

148

TABLE 35

Length of Stay
by Place of Death

Length of Stay in Months	Total %	#	Place of Death Home %	Other %
Total Number	(149)		(98)	(51)
Total Percentage	100.1		100.0	100.2
Less than 1/2 month	.7	(1)	--	2.0
1/2 to 1 mo.	43.0	(64)	43.9	41.2
1 to 2 mos.	26.2	(39)	25.5	27.5
2 to 4 mos.	14.1	(21)	12.2	17.7
Over 4 mos.	16.1	(24)	18.4	11.8

NOTES:

Percentages may not total 100.0% due to rounding.

This table excludes those persons (12.4% of total) for whom there was no answer on the question regarding place of death.

TABLE 36

Total Number of Visits
by Place of Death

Total Visits	Total		Place of Death	
			Home	Other
Total Number	(149)		(98)	(51)
Total Percentage	100.0		100.1	100.0
	%	#	%	%
None	2.7	(4)	4.1	--
1-9	40.3	(60)	34.7	51.0
10-19	27.5	(41)	27.6	27.5
20-29	16.1	(24)	17.4	13.7
30 or more	13.4	(20)	16.3	7.8

NOTES:
   This table excludes those patients (12.4%)
for whom there was no information regarding
place of death.
   Percentages may not total 100.0% due to
rounding.

TABLE 37

Total Visit Hours
by Place of Death

| Total Hours | Total | | Place of Death | |
			Home	Other
Total Number	(149)		(98)	(51)
Total Percentage	100.1		100.1	100.0
	%	#	%	%
None	3.4	(5)	4.1	2.0
1-9	49.7	(74)	43.9	60.8
10-19	24.2	(36)	25.5	21.6
20-29	11.4	(17)	13.3	7.8
30 or more	11.4	(17)	13.3	7.8

NOTES:
  Percentages may not total 100.0% due to rounding.
  This table excludes those persons (12.4%) for whom there was no information regarding place of death.

TABLE 38

Place of Death by Health
of Primary Care Person

| Place of Death | Total | | Health of PCP | |
			Poor to Fair	Good
Total Number	(137)		(44)	(93)
Total Percentage	100.0		100.0	100.0
	%	#	%	%
Home	64.2	(88)	70.5	61.3
Other	35.8	(49)	29.5	38.7

NOTE: This table excludes those persons (19.4%) for whom there was no information regarding place of death or health of primary care person.

TABLE 39

Total Number of Visits
by Sex of Patient

Total Visits	Total		Male	Female
			Sex	
Total Number	(170)		(74)	(96)
Total Percentage	100.1		100.0	100.1
	%	#	%	%
None	2.4	(4)	2.7	2.1
1-9	39.4	(67)	32.4	44.8
10-19	27.7	(47)	28.4	27.1
20-29	14.7	(25)	18.9	11.5
30 or more	15.9	(27)	17.6	14.6

NOTE: Percentages may not total 100.0% due to rounding.

TABLE 40

Total Number of Visits by Socioeconomic Status

Total Visits	Total		I	II	III	IV	V
					Hollingshead Classification		
Total Number	(125)		(3)	(10)	(18)	(57)	(37)
Total Percentage	100.0		100.0	100.0	100.0	100.0	100.0
	%	#	%	%	%	%	%
None	1.6	(2)	--	--	5.6	1.8	--
1-9	40.8	(51)	33.3	40.0	44.4	36.8	46.0
10-19	26.4	(33)	66.7	30.0	22.2	22.8	29.7
20-29	15.2	(19)	--	20.0	11.1	19.3	10.8
30 or more	16.0	(20)	--	10.0	16.7	19.3	13.5

NOTES:

On the Hollingshead scale the numeral I represents the highest social class (in terms of occupation and education) and V represents the lowest.

This table excludes those persons (26.5%) for whom there was no information concerning Hollingshead class.

154

TABLE 41

Total Number of Visits by Status at Admission

| Total Visits | Total | | | Status at Admission | | |
			Ambulatory	Bedridden	Other
Total Number	(162)		(76)	(64)	(22)
Total Percentage	100.0		99.9	100.1	100.0
	%	#	%	%	%
None	2.5	(4)	1.3	4.7	--
1-9	39.5	(64)	27.6	56.3	31.8
10-19	26.5	(43)	26.3	23.4	36.4
20-29	14.8	(24)	18.4	14.1	4.6
30 or more	16.7	(27)	26.3	1.6	27.3

NOTES:

Percentages may not total 100.0% due to rounding.

This table excludes those persons (4.7%) for whom there was no information regarding status at admission.

155

TABLE 42

Total Number of Visits by Health of Primary Care Person

Total Visits	Total		Health of PCP Poor to Fair	Good
Total Number	(154)		(51)	(103)
Total Percentage	100.0		100.0	100.0
	%	#	%	%
None	2.0	(3)	2.0	1.9
1-9	39.6	(61)	37.2	40.8
10-19	27.3	(42)	29.4	26.2
20-29	14.9	(23)	17.7	13.6
30 or more	16.2	(25)	13.7	17.5

NOTE: This table excludes those persons (9.4%) for whom there was no information regarding health of primary care person.

between patient status upon admission to the Hospice Home Care program and total visits. In table 41, it can be seen that patients who are bedridden at time of admission receive fewer visits than do those who are ambulatory or who are ambulatory with assistance. Data from table 55 would indicate the reason for this relationship: bedridden patients have a much shorter length of stay, because they die sooner than do the ambulatory patients.

No relationship was found between the number of visits and the health of the primary care person, which points to the question of how care-givers in poor health cope with the needs of the dying person (table 42).

As one might suspect a statistically significant relationship was found between the number of months on the Hospice program and visit hours and total visits (tables not shown). The number of visits tends to increase the longer a person is on the program; the same is true for visit hours.

Total visits were related to various aspects associated with the primary care person. No statistically significant relationship was found between total visits and the number of persons in the household, the age of the primary care person, or whether additional support came from family members or from other persons. The same is true of the relationship between total visits and patient age, marital status, race, education, awareness of diagnosis, and pain experienced.

Awareness of Diagnosis

Tables 43 and 44 portray relationships between whether the patient was aware of the diagnosis and selected patient characteristics.

The relationship between patient age and awareness of diagnosis is shown in table 43.

157

TABLE 43

Patient Awareness of Diagnosis by Age at Admission

Aware of Diagnosis	Total	Less than 30	30-49	50-59	Age at Admission 60-69	70-79	80 and over
Total Number	157	2	18	29	61	34	13
Total Percentage	100.0	100.0	99.9	100.0	100.0	100.0	100.1
	%	%	%	%	%	%	%
Yes	73.9	100.0	94.4	75.9	73.8	70.6	46.2
No	26.1	--	5.6	24.1	26.2	29.4	53.9

NOTES:

Percentages may not total 100.0% due to rounding.
This table excludes those people (7.7% of total) for whom no information was
recorded regarding awareness of diagnosis.

158

TABLE 44

Patient Awareness of Diagnosis by Level of Education

Aware of Diagnosis	Total		More than High School	High School Graduate	Less than High School
			Level of Education		
Total Number	(142)		(30)	(47)	(65)
Total Percentage	100.0		100.0	100.0	100.0
	%	#	%	%	%
Yes	73.9	(105)	83.3	89.4	58.5
No	26.1	(37)	16.7	10.6	41.5

NOTE: This table excludes those persons (16.5%) for whom there were missing data concerning level of education or awareness of diagnosis.

159

The association is statistically significant (p = 0.05), indicating that young persons are more aware of the diagnosis than are those in the older age groups.

A statistically significant relationship was also found between awareness of diagnosis and the educational level attained by the patient. As shown in table 44, those who are not high school graduates are markedly less aware of their diagnosis (p = 0.0005).

No statistical significance was found between awareness of diagnosis and other attributes studied (tables not shown). These included patient occupation, sex, marital status, race, ethnic background, religion, social class, source of payment, pain, number of months in the Hospice program, number of persons in the household, and relationship of primary care persons.

Pain

Tables 45 to 51 focus on the relationship between selected variables and whether the patient complained of pain upon admission to the Hospice Home Care program.

Table 45 shows the relationship between occupation and pain at admission to the program. A greater percentage of blue collar workers reported pain than did white collar workers.

No statistically significant relationships were discovered between the incidence of pain and when the patient last worked (table 46). However, the proportion of patients reporting pain tends to decrease the longer patients are out of work.

Table 47 shows that those in Class V complained of more pain than the other classes. No statistically significant relationships were found between pain and religion (table 48) and whether the patient practiced religion (table 49).

Table 50 shows the relationship between pain at admission and length of stay in the program. No statistically significant relationship was found between the patient's complaint of pain at time of admission and number of months in the program. Table 51 shows no difference in the place of death when related to incidence of pain on admission to the program.

No statistically significant relationships were found between pain and age of patient, sex, marital status, patient educational level, race, or ethnic background (tables not shown).

Primary Care Person's Relationship to Patient

Table 52 shows a statistically significant relationship (p = 0.00012) between sex of the patient and the relationship of the primary care-giver to the patient. Male patients are more apt than females to have their spouses as the primary care person, whereas more females than males were cared for by children.

Number of Months as a Patient in the Hospice Home Care Program

The number of months a person remains as a Hospice patient (length of stay) is related to selected variables in tables 53-55. No statistically significant relationships were found between length of stay and age (table 53); sex (table 54); or marital status, education, occupation, when last worked, race, religion, whether the patient practiced religion, or social class (tables not shown).

161

TABLE 45

Incidence of Pain
by Occupation

Incidence of Pain	Total		Occupation White Collar	Blue Collar
Total Number	(154)		(61)	(93)
Total Percentage	100.0		100.0	100.0
	%	#	%	%
Pain	65.6	(101)	59.0	69.9
No Pain	34.4	(53)	41.0	30.1

NOTE: This table excludes those persons (9.4% of total) for whom there was no answer on the question regarding occupation.

TABLE 46

Incidence of Pain by When Last Worked

Incidence of Pain	Total		1 Year or Less Ago	When Last Worked More than 1 Year Ago	Never Worked
Total Number	(137)		(52)	(61)	(24)
Total Percentage	100.0		100.0	100.0	100.0
	%	#	%	%	%
Pain	67.2	(92)	73.1	68.9	50.0
No pain	32.8	(45)	26.9	31.1	50.0

NOTE: This table excludes those persons (19.4% of total) for whom there was no answer to the question regarding date last worked.

TABLE 47

Incidence of Pain by Socioeconomic Status

Incidence of Pain	Total		Hollingshead Classification				
			I	II	III	IV	V
Total Number	(125)		(3)	(10)	(18)	(57)	(37)
Total Percentage	100.0		100.0	100.0	100.0	100.0	100.0
	%	#	%	%	%	%	%
Pain	70.4	(88)	66.7	70.0	66.7	63.2	83.8
No pain	29.6	(37)	33.3	30.0	33.3	36.8	16.2

NOTES:

On the Hollingshead scale the numeral I represents the highest social class (in terms of occupation and education) and V represents the lowest.

This table excludes those persons (32.4% of total) for whom there was no recorded Hollingshead classification.

164

TABLE 48

Incidence of Pain by Religion

Incidence of Pain	Total		Protestant	Religion Catholic	Other
Total Number	(165)		(38)	(111)	(16)
Total Percentage	100.0		100.0	100.0	100.1
	%	#	%	%	%
Pain	67.3	(111)	57.9	68.5	81.3
No pain	32.7	(54)	42.1	31.5	18.8

NOTES:

Percentages may not total 100.0% due to rounding.
This table excludes those persons (2.9% of total) for whom there was no answer on the question regarding religion.

165

TABLE 49

Incidence of Pain by
Whether Practicing Religion

Incidence of Pain	Total		Practicing	Non-Practicing
Total Number	(160)		(131)	(29)
Total Percentage	100.0		100.0	100.0
	%	#	%	%
Pain	67.5	(108)	66.4	72.4
No pain	32.5	(52)	33.6	27.6

NOTE: This table excludes those persons (5.9% of total) for whom there was no answer on the question regarding practice of religion.

TABLE 50

Length of Stay by
Incidence of Pain

Length of Stay in Months	Total		Incidence of Pain	
			Pain	No Pain
Total Number	(170)		(113)	(57)
Total Percentage	100.0		100.0	100.0
	%	#	%	%
Less than 1/2 mo.	8.2	(14)	8.0	8.8
1/2 to 1 mo.	37.7	(64)	34.5	43.9
1 to 2 mos.	23.5	(40)	26.5	17.5
2 to 4 mos.	12.4	(21)	13.3	10.5
Over 4 mos.	18.2	(31)	17.7	19.3

TABLE 51

Incidence of Pain
by Place of Death

Incidence of Pain	Total		Place of Death Home	Other
Total Number	(149)		(98)	(51)
Total Percentage	100.0		100.1	100.0
	%	#	%	%
Pain	67.1	(100)	67.4	66.7
No Pain	32.9	(49)	32.7	33.3

NOTES:
  Percentages may not total 100.0% due to rounding.
  This table excludes those persons (12.4%) for whom there was no information regarding place of death.

TABLE 52

Relationship of Primary Care Person
to Patient by Sex of Patient

Relationship of Primary Care Person to Patient	Total		Sex	
			Male	Female
Total Number	(168)		(74)	(94)
Total Percentage	100.0		100.0	100.0
	%	#	%	%
Spouse	58.9	(99)	74.3	46.8
Child	22.6	(38)	12.2	30.9
Other	18.5	(31)	13.5	22.3

NOTE: This table excludes those persons (1.2% of total) for whom no relationship of primary care person was recorded.

TABLE 53

Length of Stay by Age of Patient

Length of Stay	Total		Under 30	30-49	Age of Patient 50-59	60-69	70-79	80 and over
	%	#						
Total Number	(170)		(2)	(20)	(31)	(66)	(37)	(14)
Total Percentage	100.0		100.0	100.0	100.0	100.0	99.9	100.0
	%		%	%	%	%	%	%
Less than 1/2 mo.	8.2	(14)	50.0	5.0	6.5	4.6	16.2	7.1
1/2 to 1 month	37.7	(64)	--	35.0	41.9	43.9	29.7	28.6
1 to 2 months	23.5	(40)	--	30.0	22.6	21.2	24.3	28.6
2 to 4 months	12.4	(21)	--	15.0	9.7	13.6	8.1	21.4
Over 4 months	18.2	(31)	50.0	15.0	19.4	16.7	21.6	14.3

NOTE: Percentages may not total 100.0% due to rounding.

170

TABLE 54

Length of Stay
by Sex of Patient

| Length | | | Sex | |
of Stay	Total		Male	Female
Total Number	(170)		(74)	(96)
Total Percentage	100.0		100.1	100.0
	%	#	%	%
Less than 1/2 mo.	8.2	(14)	9.5	7.3
1/2 to 1 mo.	37.7	(64)	33.8	40.6
1 to 2 mos.	23.5	(40)	28.4	19.8
2 to 4 mos.	12.4	(21)	14.9	10.4
Over 4 mos.	18.2	(31)	13.5	21.9

NOTE: Percentages may not total 100.0% due to rounding.

TABLE 55

Length of Stay by Status at Admission

Length of Stay	Total		Status at Admission		
			Ambulatory	Bedridden	Other
Total Number	(162)		(76)	(64)	(22)
Total Percentage	100.0		100.1	100.1	100.1
	%	#	%	%	%
Less than 1/2 mo.	8.6	(14)	11.8	6.3	4.6
1/2 to 1 mo.	37.0	(60)	21.1	57.8	31.8
1 to 2 mos.	23.5	(38)	21.1	25.0	27.3
2 to 4 mos.	12.4	(20)	17.1	4.7	18.2
Over 4 mos.	18.5	(30)	29.0	6.3	18.2

NOTES:

Percentages may not total 100.0% due to rounding.

This table excludes those persons (4.7% of total) for whom there was no information regarding status at admission.

172

A statistically significant relationship
(p = 0.0001) was found between length of stay in
the Hospice Home Care program and the patient's
status at admission. As table 55 shows, patients
who are ambulatory at admission have longer
lengths of stay and patients who are bedridden
at admission have shorter lengths of stay.

The relationship between length of stay and
certain variables dealing with the patient's
home environment and the primary care person was
examined. No statistically significant
relationships were found between length of stay
and the number of persons in the patient's
household; whether the primary care person was
the patient's spouse, child, or some other
person; and the age, sex, or health status of
the primary care person (tables not shown).

Summary of Staff Activities

Table 56 provides some insight into Hospice
staff activity during the period of the study.
All data are presented on the basis of "per
person per month."

On the average each staff member performed
26.1 visits per month. These visits took, on
the average, 28.7 hours total, and staff spent
an average of 11.7 hours per month in travel
time, yielding a total of 40.6 hours per month
in visiting patients.

The greatest proportion of visits made by
Hospice Home Care personnel was for ongoing
assessment, 17.9 visits on average; second in
line were friendly supportive visits, 12.1 on
average.

Among all types of personnel, volunteers
had the highest average number of total visits
(46.9); social workers had the least (10.2).

173

TABLE 56

Summary of Hospice Staff Activities
per Person per Month

Type of Activity	All Personnel	Mean LPN	RN	MD	SW	Vol.
Total Visits	26.1	23.7	32.8	12.3	10.2	46.9
Total visit hours	28.7	24.5	31.2	9.4	8.9	86.9
Travel time	11.7	9.7	13.9	5.3	3.2	28.1
Total time	40.6	34.1	44.7	14.6	12.1	119.1
Initial assessment visit	2.3	1.9	2.4	1.6	2.6	--
Ongoing assessment visit	17.9	16.0	23.9	2.8	2.5	2.7
Direct physical care visit	7.1	3.5	9.1	1.0	--	7.4
Treat. physical care visit	3.1	2.4	3.4	1.0	--	--
Medication physical care visit	3.3	2.5	3.9	1.0	--	--
Counseling supportive care	8.2	5.3	11.3	1.5	4.9	5.5
Teaching supportive care visit	6.4	4.6	7.4	1.0	1.0	--
Friendly supportive care	12.1	6.6	8.6	2.0	2.0	37.7

Physician supervision visit	2.5	1.0	1.0	4.0	--	--
Nurse supervision visit	1.6	2.0	1.5	--	--	--
Volunteer supervision visit	3.8	2.4	5.0	2.0	--	2.5
Agency supervision visit	1.0	1.0	1.0	--	--	--
Transportation visit	6.8	1.0	1.2	--	1.0	11.6
Bereavement visit	3.9	3.5	4.4	2.0	4.3	2.3
Physician consultation	8.1	--	--	8.1	--	--
Physician chemotherapy	1.5	--	--	1.5	--	--
Physician symptom control	6.8	--	--	6.8	--	--
Death pronouncement	1.7	1.3	1.3	2.3	--	--
Discharges	1.4	--	1.7	1.3	--	--

This pattern holds true also for total visit hours, travel time, and total time. Clearly, volunteer personnel are significant contributors to Hospice Home Care activities.

Among all types of personnel, registered nurses made the most ongoing assessment visits (23.9) and also made the most direct physical care visits (9.1). On the average, physicians made 4.0 visits that included physician supervision.

In general, most LPN time on visits was spent in ongoing assessments and in providing friendly supportive care and counseling. Registered nurses spent most of their efforts in ongoing assessment visits, followed by counseling and direct physical care visits. Physician time was spent mostly in physician consultation followed by symptom control and supervision. Social workers were more apt to spend their time in counseling and supportive care, and in bereavement visits. Volunteers were spending most of their effort in friendly supportive care visits, transportation visits, and direct physical care visits.

Considering all personnel associated with patient home care visits, volunteers spent the most time (119.1 hours per month), followed by registered nurses (44.7), licensed practical nurses (34.1), physicians (14.6), and social workers (12.1 hours per month).

Part III
The Evaluation Study

CHAPTER 9

Terminal Care: Review of the Literature

The Hospice program has evolved in part as an attempt to compensate for the inadequacies of the present medical system, acute-care hospitals, and physicians in relieving the physical distress of the terminal cancer patient. At present in our society, there is slim prospect that the average terminal patient suffering from pain will find complete relief. Analgesic dosages are generally standardized and are seldom calibrated to meet the patient's individual needs; scheduling of pain-relieving medications is also seldom suited to the patient's requirements. The patient is thus often sentenced to pass through consecutive stages of sedation, uneasiness, and intense suffering. Narcotics prescribed to be given when needed (prn--pro re nata) are often withheld by members of the medical staff to avoid addicting the patient and they are seldom administered before the patient is in a state of acute distress.[1]

THE PROBLEM OF PAIN

The findings in studies by John Hinton[2] and C. M. Saunders[3] that the terminal cancer patient's physical distress is inadequately controlled in the acute-care or general hospital has been borne out in a study of terminal care by Dr. Richard Lamerton,[4] who discovered that one-fifth of all hospitalized terminal cancer patients are in severe pain. Yet, the situation may be far worse if the patient chooses to die at home. Researchers at the Marie Curie Foundation in 1952 found that 68 percent of patients with cancer who were being cared for at home experienced moderate to severe suffering.[5] Similarly Dewi Rees, a family practitioner, found that 44 percent of his dying patients being cared for at home were suffering continuous pain despite his efforts.[6]

The failure to reduce pain has not, however, been universal. Accounts of the accomplishments of the staff at St. Christopher's Hospice in London contrast markedly with the stated results of other efforts at pain control. In a study of 1,500 patients admitted to St. Christopher's for treatment, it was found that 99 percent of patients with severe pain at the time of their admission were afforded relief. Dr. Lamerton has suggested that the pain experienced by those being cared for at home could be sharply reduced by introducing a Hospice Home Care team and outpatient clinic into the patient's total care regimen. In his view, the terminal patient is more efficiently and properly cared for under Hospice guidance than in the general hospital or by the family practitioner at home.[7] This is due in part to the willingness of Hospice staff to recognize the various influences on a patient's perception of pain. Dr. Cicely Saunders maintains that in addition to the pain caused directly by the malignancy, cancer patients are subject to pain from symptoms that are byproducts of the disease or treatment. Moreover, the patient's perception and experience of pain are strongly influenced by emotional responses.[8] Relief of pain in the terminally ill is thus a multi-faceted problem: attention must be given to the physical pain, the perception of the sensation, and the patient's emotional reaction to it.

Dr. Saunders notes that an expression of interest in each patient's particular problems may eliminate much physical distress. The presence of a caring figure who listens and attempts to understand the sensation of pain that the patient is experiencing is perhaps one of the most important factors in the relief of that pain.[9] This contention is supported by Kubler-Ross,[10] Hinton,[11] and Lamerton,[12] who concur that the presence of someone who spends time visiting and listening to the patient is a fundamental need of the terminally ill. However, according to Rabin and Rabin, health care professionals seek to avoid being in the presence of the dying.[13] R. W. Buckingham reported that dying patients are often relegated to back rooms where they are left alone and ignored for extended periods of time.[14] There is a general tendency for members of the medical and nursing staff to avoid eye contact and to limit interaction with dying patients to brief, task-oriented episodes. Physicians make perfunctory and hasty rounds, frequently in groups of twos and threes, thereby intimidating the patient and eliminating opportunities for communication.[15] Hackett and Weisman observed that when the patient suffering a malignancy is found to be incurable, the physician commonly requests that the chaplain make regular visits and subsequently withdraws.[16] Because of such general avoidance of dying patients by health care personnel, treatment of the emotional dimensions of pain is usually neglected.[17] The consequences of such neglect are compounded by the special problems of chronic pain.

Nature of Chronic Pain

Chronic pain is perpetual and progressive rather than transient and reversible, the characteristics of acute pain. Physical, psychological, interpersonal, financial, and spiritual factors are the major components of chronic pain, and the complex interaction of these factors leads to what Saunders has termed "total pain."[18] Such pain appears to be meaningless and, because it occurs as an adjunct to advanced malignant disease, often forcibly reminds the patient of the terminal prognosis, thereby intensifying distress. The terminal patient's anticipation of extended episodes of pain leads to anxiety, depression, and insomnia, and these in turn aggravate physical pain.[19] In addition, other physical problems such as bedsores, constipation, cystitis, and musculoskeletal problems, although not a consequence of malignancy, tend to occur concomitantly with the malignant process. Effective relief of a terminal patient's discomfort therefore calls for the efforts of an interdisciplinary team in delivering proper nursing care.

The first step in attempting to alleviate

a patient's pain is to ascertain the individual's particular nursing needs. Education of the patient and his family in the aspects of nursing care that the patient will require is of basic importance in providing him with optimal comfort.[20] Frequent changes in position are required for the bedridden to prevent bedsores; proper dietary habits must be introduced to prevent constipation or gastro-intestinal distress; limited exercise is advisable for the nonambulatory to prevent the onset of musculoskeletal pain, and for the ambulatory to ensure that they maintain maximum mobility. Many of the discomforts that are common symptoms of malignant disease can be mitigated. Anorexia may be alleviated by the use of glucocortico-steroids and attention to the patient's dietary preferences. Intractable vomiting or nausea, whether due to potent narcotic analgesic intake, tumorous obstruction, bleeding from a cancerous growth, biochemical upset, or pressure on the gastrointestinal tract, may be meliorated by administration of an antiemetic. Dysphagia may be relieved with application of local anesthetics and careful assistance to the patient in drinking cool fluids. Similarly, dehydration, hiccups, itching, insomnia, urinary complications, and fungating growths should not plague the dying patient if prompt and effective relief can be provided.[21]

When pain cannot be alleviated through nursing techniques alone, and when diversions such as occupational therapy, physical therapy, entertainment, and mild forms of recreation are to no avail, analgesic agents may be needed.[22] Nonnarcotic analgesics such as aspirin and Tylenol may be quite effective and are the substances most likely to be initially pre-scribed for pain relief. If the nonnarcotics

183

prove insufficient in controlling the pain, the patient is often transferred onto a synthetic narcotic analgesic. Nausea and vomiting, especially with patients in the advanced stages of cancer, are commonly associated with the use of narcotics. To counteract such side effects, an antiemetic is usually prescribed concurrently.

If the patient's pain becomes so severe that synthetic narcotics fail to provide sufficient analgesia, the Hospice physician may prescribe morphine in the United States or diamorphine in the United Kingdom. Caution is urged in the use of narcotic analgesics, and many physicians and medical sources have issued warnings concerning the danger of tolerance, addiction, and diminishing awareness in the patient. However, Dr. R. G. Twycross, in an effort to moderate physicians' common fears of the effects of narcotic analgesics, has documented much positive clinical experience in the use of narcotic analgesics at St. Christopher's Hospice. To determine whether narcotic analgesia led to the impairment of mental faculties or the development of tolerance or addiction, Twycross observed 500 patients consecutively admitted to the Hospice with advanced malignant disease. He concluded that drowsiness and detachment from reality are related more to advanced physical disability than to a particular narcotic dosage.[23] Twycross also concluded that the necessity for increasing narcotic dosages is caused more by increased pain than by tolerance; most upward adjustments in diamorphine dosage were for pain associated with different metastatic lesions. With oral administration of morphine, as in the Brompton narcotic mixture prescribed by Hospice physicians, dependence develops less rapidly and possibly to a lesser degree.[24] Dr. Lack describes how to titrate the level of analgesia against the degree of pain experienced by the patient, increasing the dosage gradually until the pain is alleviated. The subsequent dose is given before the effects of the previous dose have subsided, thus keeping pain in abeyance.[25]

Nonetheless, the majority of physicians who care for the terminally ill fear addiction, tolerance, and mental impairment in their patients and consequently prescribe narcotics on a four-hourly prn or "as needed/when necessary" basis. Under this system of narcotic administration the patient must be in pain before he is able to receive the drug; if the therapeutic regimen calls for pain-killers every four hours and he demonstrates a need for pain-relieving medication before that time has elapsed, he is left to suffer out the remaining interval in pain.

Aims of Treatment of Pain

According to B. M. Mount, there are several aims in treating the intractable pain of advanced cancer.[26] Clarification of the cause of the pain is an essential first aim in symptom control and may suggest possible modes of therapeutic intervention. Awareness of the cause of the pain and of the existence of effective therapies for its relief serves to remove the patient from the characteristic state of meaningless helplessness and hopelessness described by LeShan.[27] A second important aim is the prevention of pain, as opposed to treatment once pain has occurred. Repeated success at pre-venting pain lessens the anxious anticipation and memory of pain, and frequently the amount of analgesic required for the maintenance of comfort decreases.[28]

Another aim in treatment is to bring about a pain-free state without sedation. Many patients feel that their only alternatives are constant pain or perpetual somnolence. Comfort and an unclouded sensorium can be achieved simultaneously, however, if the analgesic dosage is carefully regulated to the individual's needs.[29] Patients need to be able to relate to environment in a normal manner--neither euphoric due to an excess of drugs nor distressed due to inadequate medication. Even the mode of administration should be considered in terms of the maximum benefit to the patient: Oral analgesia allows the patient a degree of mobility and independence not afforded by parenteral administration.[30]

There is convincing evidence that the Brompton mixture, an oral narcotic preparation given with a phenothiazine, effectively controls severe pain. The mixture is used when milder narcotic and nonnarcotic preparations prove ineffective. Yet, despite its potent analgesic effects, the mixture may be used for many months and even several years without dose escalation.[31] Moreover, according to R. Melzack et al., the Brompton mixture has a strong effect on the sensory, affective, and evaluative dimensions of pain as well as on its physical component.[32] In a study of the effects of the Brompton mixture at McGill University in Montreal, researchers found that the psychological benefit of the supportive environment provided in a palliative care unit combined with the analgesic effects of the narcotic medication together provided optimal pain relief.[33]

In addition to the effective use of analgesics, the staff at St. Christopher's employs other palliative measures such as radio-therapy, hormone therapy, and surgical relief of symptoms due to tumorous pressure. Through an understanding of chronic pain and the proper use of medication, nursing care, and diversional activity, Dr. Saunders and the staff at St. Christopher's have found that much of the pain of cancer is not an inevitable consequence of the disease, but is capable of being meliorated if a willingness to depart from traditional medical practices exists.[34]

ANXIETY AND DEPRESSION

In recent years, efforts have been made by Elisabeth Kubler-Ross,[35] John Hinton,[36] Colin Murray Parkes,[37] and others to discern the reactions of dying patients to their terminal illness and imminent death. Observations have focused on the patients' thoughts, fears, and desires. In one such effort a controlled trial was employed to investigate the mental and physical distress of dying patients, comparing patients dying from various carcinomas with patients who were seriously, although not fatally, ill with diseases of comparable organs. A substantially greater degree of anxiety and depression was found in the dying patients, with the greatest degree occurring in those dying patients under age 50 with young, dependent children.[38]

The prospect of death is a source of profound fear for many people and as Colin Murray Parkes found, such fear increases the anxiety and depression suffered by the dying patient.[39] Fear of death and dying may relate to a host of factors: separation from family, home, and job; inability to complete a major life task or responsibility; guilt at leaving dependents behind and concern over the unforeseen consequences of such perceived abandonment.

187

In addition, the loss of control over bodily functions and the attendant necessity for reliance on others, mutilation and pain, existence as a nuisance to loved ones, unpreparedness for death and uncertainty concerning what it holds in store--all these factors combine to precipitate depression.[40]

John Hinton maintains that the incidence of anxiety is greater among those who experience a long terminal illness than among those whose illness is relatively brief. In addition, young people are characteristically more anxious during the course of a fatal disease than are the elderly.[41] Williams and Cole have reported that those who are highly religious have a considerably lower degree of anxiety and apprehension about death than do less religious patients.[42] The degree of anxiety that one experiences may in turn be exacerbated by disfigurement and physical distress. It is especially aggravated in those persons suffering from difficult breathing. Such findings reflect the personal impact of those inevitable concomitants of terminal disease which Hinton perceives as causative agents in depression among the fatally ill. Discomfort, physical deterioration, the realization that life is ending, and the individual's characteristic manner of coping with the exigencies of life will all determine the degree and nature of the depression experienced by that patient.[43]

Although pain, weight loss, and other manifestations of physical deterioration are a source of great distress to the dying person, coping with the social and emotional issues of imminent death is often of even greater concern to the patient. It is, therefore, imperative that the research on the emotional needs of the dying continue. There is general agreement at present as to the importance of open

188

communication and trust between patient, physician, and other health care personnel. The part such interactions play in lending support to the patient must be explored, maximized, and reinforced.

Stages of Psychological Reaction

Dr. Kubler-Ross has recorded her experience in observing and learning from dying patients in case studies and impressions. In reviewing the anxieties, fears, and hopes of those patients with whom she shared time and psychotherapeutic relations during the final stages of life, Kubler-Ross noted that, despite the idiosyncratic nature of each individual's dying process, patients generally seem to pass through relatively distinct phases of psychological reaction.[44]

The first stage is characterized by denial and isolation. The typical attitude assumed by the person at this time is: "No, not me." This stage serves to cushion the psychic trauma posed by imminent extinction. Some people, Kubler-Ross noted, never move beyond this point of denial.

The second stage is one of anger. When the person can no longer maintain the defenses of denial and lets go of the artificial images of health and well-being which have sustained him through the initial shock, denial is replaced by feelings of anger, hostility, envy, and resentment. The all-consuming question is: "Why me?" Overwhelmed by the inequity of this fate, the patient wonders bitterly why such catastrophe did not befall someone else. Eager to vent his hostility, he searches for grievances. As a consequence his anger, sometimes unreasonable, is often directed toward family, friends, and the medical and nursing staff charged with his care.

The third stage is described as one of bargaining with God or nature. In this stage the patient attempts to manipulate his fate by bartering good behavior for modest wishes. His wish is most often for a brief extension of life, perhaps to live through an important event such as the marriage of a child. Another frequent wish is for a few days free of pain and physical discomfort. Kubler-Ross points out that such bargaining is normal and natural and should be regarded as preparation for the ultimate acceptance of one's approaching death.[45]

When the terminal patient begins to decline in strength, when he is no longer overtly healthy and is confronted with the possibility of further hospitalizations, his initial resilience, stoicism, and anger give way to a profound sense of loss. This is the fourth stage, the stage of depression. At this time the patient withdraws into himself to cope with the many losses facing him. He becomes acutely aware of his approaching death, especially insofar as it promises permanent loss and separation, and grieves in response. Kubler-Ross differentiates this depression into two different types requiring different treatment: reactive and preparatory. Reactive depression is precipitated by one of the many attendant problems and losses of terminal illness. The patient may be concerned because the cost of his illness is draining financial reserves from his survivors. A parent may be worried about who will care for his or her children. Loss of health, attractiveness, time, freedom, and mobility, especially among hospitalized patients--all these separation experiences activate grief.[46]

Preparatory depression is not a reaction to past or present loss, but an anticipation of

190

impending losses. In this state the patient regards death as a triple separation: separation from body, separation from community and loved ones, and separation from earthly possessions. The depression itself may be a tool to prepare the dying person for the imminent loss of all in life that is dear to him, in order to facilitate the state of acceptance. If he is allowed to feel and contemplate his sorrow, such final acceptance will be easier; the encouragement and reassurance so helpful in dealing with reactive depression are therefore contraindicated here. Silent support and cooperation are all that are needed to assist the patient in his passage through this beneficial and normal state of reorganization and emotional preparation. For the patient to die in a stage of acceptance and peace he must work through his anguish and anxieties. As Porter has phrased it, he must give himself "permission to die."[47]

If the patient has had adequate time and perhaps some assistance in working through the previous four stages he may reach a stage free of anger, resentment, and depression. He will have mourned his losses to come and prepared himself to await his death with peaceful expectation. This is the stage of acceptance toward which Kubler-Ross asserts the doctor should direct his plan of psychological management.

The five phases outlined by Kubler-Ross, although implicitly successive, do not form a rigid sequence of predictable states through which every patient characteristically and uniformly passes. The process of dying is as personal and unique as the process of living. Each person reacts in a manner that is exclusively his own. Each patient will progress at his own pace in his own individual fashion:

perhaps returning periodically from one stage to a previous stage, perhaps passing quickly to a state of ready acceptance, perhaps remaining in the stage of denial up through the very end.

In a study conducted by R. J. Carey, the most frequently expressed concern among dying patients was the fear of being a burden to others.[48] Sigmund Kahn maintains that potential desertion, the attendant fear of terminal dependence, is the major problem faced by the dying.[49] Such concerns, together with fear of separation from loved ones and of adverse consequences for those left behind, illustrate the need for unfaltering professional support on behalf of both patient and family through the social crises that arise.

Arnold Rosin has asserted that the common conceptual model of illness, represented by an equation in which the prognosis for life and activity is equal to the product of the diagnosis and the response to treatment, is inadequate because it excludes other determinants of the quality of life. Rosin maintains that the psychological makeup of the individual and his emotional response to terminal illness combine to influence the patient's qualitative prognosis (as distinct from survival time).[50] Yet, the effects of a patient's emotional reaction and previous life experience on his symptomatic response are often not considered when prescribing treatment. Excessive weight is given to the impact of the pathological process alone. Medical personnel must observe the process of dying as well as the course of the malignancy in assessing the results of treatment in the terminally ill. An increased sense of well-being and improved functioning in a terminal patient might not be the consequence of specific treatment of the disease. Similarly, failure to improve may not indicate inadequate therapy.

Many researchers in the field of pain relief have pointed out that the individual's characteristic reaction to pain largely determines both the course of the disease and degree of pain experienced. Indeed, according to Colin Murray Parkes, the way in which a person reacts to his illness may even prolong his life.[51] Pain, in turn, can cause the emergence of depression or hostility. Such affective-reactive interaction dictates the need for personal attention in the care of the dying and the need to elucidate the fears regarding death in relation to the symptoms and emotions of dying patients. Establishment of a personal rapport with the dying patient is a prerequisite to fully understanding the patient's clinical progress. The effects of such personal contact, pain control, familial support, and proper nursing care are most certainly synergistic.

The care of terminally ill patients should enable them to maintain their abilities to function and to contribute as full human beings. Unfortunately, these goals are often impossible to achieve in present institutional settings. The structure, organization, and philosophy of the medical staff in acute-care hospitals are geared toward aggressive, curative intervention. Characteristically such facilities exclude certain essential elements in the delivery of proper terminal care: involvement of the family in the patient's medical situation which facilitates acceptance and alleviates potential guilt; care of the patient and family with respect to all relevant needs--physical, emotional, spiritual, and social; effective use of narcotics for the abolition of pain; execution of the patient's wishes with respect to his environment and therapy; teamwork among the medical staff in order to promote the patient's total well-being.

Inadequacies of Current Care System

Those examining current practices in the care of the terminally ill generally agree that such care is usually limited, deficient, or inappropriate, and in many cases devastating to the patient. David Shephard cites three reasons for the pervasive inadequacy of terminal care.[52] First, the emphasis on investigation and treatment leads the practitioner to regard the patient as a disease entity and not as a whole person. As Kubler-Ross has illustrated, the patient "may cry for rest, peace, and dignity but he will get infusions, transfusions, a heart machine, or tracheotomy."[53] Even when beyond the stage of possible recovery, the patient is often inappropriately subjected to the rigors of curative therapy. A second deficiency in terminal care is inappropriate environment: In an acute-care hospital the orientation of facilities, policies, and staff is toward cure rather than palliation, whereas a chronic-care institution is by nature dedicated to meeting the everyday needs of its patients. Inadequate care may also be a consequence of the psychological inability of people in our society to confront the dying.[54] Ironically, investigators have found that physicians are more fearful of death than are members of any other occupation. Feifel has postulated that the practice of curative medicine facilitates and reinforces the denial of death, thereby preventing physicians from comforting their patients and from providing nonclinical, social, and personal support.[55]

The training of personnel has exacerbated rather than alleviated the widespread inability to confront or to cope with death. Dehumanizing

194

approaches to patient care result when staff
anxieties intervene in the process of assisting
the dying person. Defensive behavior such as
indifference, hostility, or detachment from the
dying person on the part of staff and friends
magnifies the loneliness of hospitalization and
accentuates withdrawal of the patient, who is
already experiencing a diminished sense of self
and decreasing awareness of environment.[56] The
pressures for efficiency and organization
demanded in the routine of hospital activities
add to the strained interaction between staff
and patient.

The tendency to forget about the patient
once he is labeled incurable elicits a dreadful
sense of desolation and loneliness and
precipitates a state of depression and intro-
version in the victim of such attitudes. He may
become overwhelmed with hopelessness, withdraw-
ing into "a dark and haunted cavern of dreams
and imaginings."[57]

The physician who avoids informing the
patient of the diagnosis and prognosis fosters
isolation, suspicion, and mistrust between
patients, families, and the medical staff. The
resultant breakdown in communication illustrates
that physicians cannot be effective in treating
the terminally ill if they focus solely on the
physiological process of death and ignore its
personal, social, spiritual, and cultural
dimensions.[58]

According to Balfour Mount, there are three
goals in the treatment of malignant disease: to
cure, to prolong life, and to palliate.[59]
Whereas extensive resources have been devoted
to attempts at curing and, secondarily, at
prolonging life, little has been done to
improve the quality of life for those to whom
the first two strategies are irrelevant. Means
must be sought to meet the special needs of

patients whose only alternative is appropriate palliative care. A change in emphasis, from curing to caring, must receive popular acceptance before proper terminal care can take hold.

THE PATIENT'S FAMILY

Little research has been done to identify the factors of greatest importance to the family of the terminal patient. Documentation of the key functions carried out through patient-family interaction would perhaps alter the perceptions of staff members who regard the presence of the family as an annoyance, and help to change hospital regulations which militate against favorable adjustments of the patient and family by excluding the family from participation in the dying process.

The physical, social, and emotional needs of both patient and family must be addressed as part of a comprehensive care program. The caring institution or team must be able constantly to shift its focus, to detect whether it is the patient, the family, or the patient-family unit which is momentarily in need of assistance in coping with the patient's state of terminal malignancy.[60] As Lamerton noticed during his experience at St. Joseph's Hospice in London, some relatives will be effective and essential components of the caring side of the team; others will be patients along with the dying family member, and others will alternately assume both roles. Some relatives will remain in the hospital overnight to deliver vigilant attention to their loved one or to be close at hand if death is imminent; others will remain because they are "too distressed to return home alone." In any case, relatives should always "be kept clearly in the picture," and to the extent that they are patients as well, relatives should be cared for along with the dying.[61] Unrestricted visiting facilitates the contribution of staff members to the well-being of the family, alleviates the patient's isolation and loneliness, and eases the family into realization of the transitions to occur with the death of one of its members.

Staff interviews with the family help the service team to gain insight into the family's manner of coping with emotions generated by the terminal malignancy of a close relative. Such knowledge is vital to the success of any effort at assisting the family through the difficult transition they must endure. Staff interviews also provide the patient and family with an opportunity to air concerns and openly confront troublesome issues which they had feared to discuss under other circumstances. Freedom to ventilate fears arising from the negative experience of a previously deceased relative, for example, can relieve the patient and family of much unnecessary anxiety.[62] The supportive climate created by an open and receptive staff enables the staff and family to exchange information that will help maintain the patient's well-being and to correct misinformation that might interfere with the patient's care or the family's peace of mind.

Just as the patient must undergo a process of realization and adjustment before coming to terms with approaching death, the family will experience transitions in learning to adapt and reconcile themselves to such profound loss. Because family members are frequently given more information about the patient's condition during the earlier stages of the malignancy, they tend to accommodate to the difficult emotional demands of the situation earlier and are there-fore ready to support the patient through the successive trials and disappointments of progressive deterioration. By virtue of their ability to postpone grief, close family members are also enabled to support the patient through increasingly difficult times. As Colin Murray Parkes asserts, family members succeed in pushing all thoughts of the future aside by focusing their energy and concern on the needs of the patient and by denying any needs of their own. As a consequence of avoiding plans for and anticipation of the period following the patient's death, the family must always undergo a realization process once the patient is gone, however lengthy the patient's illness may have been.[63]

Effects of Home Care on Family

Experiences with death have been taken from the home only to be replaced by scenes of violent and unnatural death as depicted in the media. The act of dying has become institutionalized and mechanized; people no longer die at home where relatives and children can witness their death as a natural component of life.[64] Despite the trend away from home care, the moral and spiritual gains to society of retaining death as a family event are generally accepted in theory.[65] A less obvious but extremely important function of caring for the dying patient at home is the protection afforded the survivors in the family from the hazards of bereavement, the effects of which are both social and emotional. A recent study by Rees and Lutkins indicates that a significant difference exists in the mortality experience of grieving families, dependent upon whether the patient had died at home or in the hospital. The risk of the closest relative dying within a year of bereavement was found to double if the first death had occurred in a hospital rather than at home.[66] For those cases in which the patient was cared for at home prior to death, the ability of family members to resist a devastating and prolonged period of grief is partially attributable to the continuing support of professionals who had assisted in the care of the patient and to the preparatory value of anticipatory grief.

To date, no study of the specific home care needs of patients has been reported and there has been little documentation concerning those needs and how they are most frequently met. In a retrospective examination of the experiences of 26 families who nursed a member through the terminal stages of cancer at home, the two major problems mentioned were the patient's need for physical support and lack of transportation to the hospital or clinic. Institutions often did not comply with the family's wishes for the patient's care. Some families were dismayed to find that their relative, when admitted to the hospital during the final stage of dying, was subjected to a host of exploratory tests, despite well-documented terminal malignancy. The majority of these families reported that immediate relatives or friends nursed the patient unaided by professional health workers, and only a few reported having received visiting nurse assistance.[67] Researchers have therefore not been able to distinguish whether home nursing care eases the burden of the family in meeting the expressed physical needs of the patient. However, while the patient was at home most families encountered problems severe enough to require the aid of a physician. Families regarded the medical care they received as inadequate because they received insufficient information about the patient's status, no

assistance in administering injections, and no
guidance in helping the patient to cope with
physical disintegration. The physician was
often seen as a potential source of emotional
as well as physical support, and disappointment
ensued when he failed to fulfill both roles.
Family members, equipped with neither the
knowledge nor the experience on which to base
judgment of the proper care alternative, often
express a need for education concerning certain
aspects of home care such as pain control and
diet.

The terminal illness of a family member can
be a source of physical and social as well as
emotional stress for the rest of the family.
Providing care during the night is a frequently
cited reason for loss of sleep. Outside help
in caring for the patient, either during the day
or at night, would remedy such physical strain
and help the family to give more attention and
energy to the patient's care. The additional
expenses which cancer places upon the family,
although alleviated by Medicare or Medicaid in
some instances, precipitate great financial
hardship in others. The inclusion of financial
counselors in the health care team would be a
great asset to many families for whom such
illness means being overwhelmed by unpaid bills.
In a study of 115 families with cancer patients,
the median expense for an illness of 24-months
duration was $19,054. The median income of these
families, however, was $8,000. Although health
insurance was the main source of funds, sale of
personal possessions, family loans, and life
savings were necessary to meet costs, over half
of which were attributable to physician and
hospitalization fees.[68]

Bereavement

In their study of the first year of
bereavement, Glick, Weiss, and Parkes found that
widows and widowers who were aware of the
impending deaths of their spouses suffered less
unresolved grief at the end of their first year
alone than did those who had no such fore-
warning. However, even if death of the loved
one has been anticipated for a long time and
much grieving done in advance, there is still a
resurgence of grief at the actual death.[69] The
female survivor endures bereavement much better
than her male counterpart. In addition, among
elderly people, those whose spouses succumbed
to a chronic illness of more than six months
evidence greater difficulty in adjusting during
bereavement than those who experience a shorter
period of anticipatory grief. Generally the
elderly exhibit no difference in their ability
to adjust to loss of a spouse via acute-fatal
illness as compared with death due to chronic
disease.[70] Grief over the anticipated loss of
a loved one may begin as soon as the diagnosis
is confirmed and prognosis revealed. It has
been postulated, although not confirmed
empirically, that the individual awaiting
bereavement undergoes stages similar to those
which the dying person moves through before
acceptance of his fate.

Many people react to loss by psychological
denial of the death. In such instances the
unexpressed grief tends to emerge in a severe
form triggered by a grief of lesser dimension
or an anniversary of the initial, painful loss.
Such delayed release of an earlier stress
presents itself as an excessive reaction to a
minor loss, but is indeed a painful catharsis

for the person who has never come to terms with
a great loss. Such bereavement, preceded by
suppression, can have detrimental effects on the
individual's physical and mental health,
especially when compounded by associated feelings
of anger and guilt. In such cases, proper
psychiatric management is called for to prevent
serious and prolonged social maladjustment and
to counteract any proclivity toward physical
manifestations of emotional distress.[71]
Psychiatrists, physicians, clergy, and other
bereaved persons are some of the sources of
such aid to the bereaved.

In our death-denying society, the suffering
of the bereaved is often exacerbated by the
reactions of others to his or her plight.
Loneliness due to loss of the loved one is
intensified by the failure of others to support
the survivor during the difficult period of
transition and social adjustment. People become
uncomfortable and embarrassed in the presence of
the bereaved. As if tainted by recent
experience with death, the bereaved person is
unwelcome socially. In examining the manner in
which most of Western culture stigmatizes the
bereaved, Gorer commented: "Mourning is treated
as if it were a weakness, a self-indulgence, a
reprehensible bad habit instead of a psychological necessity."[72]

Transformation of prevailing attitudes
toward and treatment of the dying would
facilitate proper adjustment of the bereaved.
When death is perceived as a natural and
necessary part of the life process,
relationships can be lived out as completely,
and terminated as productively, as possible.
It is not essential that the treatment milieu
cause the separation and anxiety of loved ones.

THE NEED FOR OBJECTIVE STUDY

Despite the emergence of a somewhat consistent philosophy of terminal care, the greatest portion of the literature on death and dying, with very few exceptions, is theoretical and anecdotal. The dearth of substantiation of current theories, the obvious need for improved care, and the pending support of many service facilities all call for documentation to provide a solid foundation for action.

Future progress in the field of terminal care will be contingent upon the accumulation of valid and reliable evaluative research data. Such data have been notably sparse and inadequate to date. Biased physician-oriented surveys and experiential commentaries comprise almost the entirety of the relevant reports. However, a few exceptional studies have recently gained recognition and may point the way for other investigations. In a study which used the technique of participant observation to explore questions concerning optimal care of dying patients and the needs of their families, Buckingham, Lack, and others compared the treatment received by terminal patients on a general surgical ward with that received on a palliative care unit.[73] Their observations supported the belief that a palliative care unit, specifically designed to meet the expressed needs of dying patients and their families, provides care for the terminally ill preferable to that received on the surgical ward. This documentation of the impact of the palliative care medical service constitutes the only extant evaluation of such a pilot project or facility in the field of terminal care.

Krant and his colleagues have begun to examine the impressions and interactions of late-stage cancer patients and their families, and to test the efficacy of specific psychosocial interventions in meeting their perceived needs.[74] Using objective measures of psychological states, Krant has considered communication regarding diagnosis, the contribution of emotional support by physicians and the clergy, depression, mood, and illness status. Although limited in scope, both the Krant and Buckingham studies mark an initial attempt to incorporate statistical criteria into the process of validation of terminal care services.

Chapter 9
NOTES

1. Erica Janzen, "Relief of Pain," _Nursing Forum_, vol. 13, no. 1 (1974).
2. John Hinton, _Dying_ (Baltimore: Penguin Books, 1974).
3. C. M. Saunders, "The Care of the Terminal Stages of Cancer," _Annals of the Royal College of Surgeons_, Supplement to vol. 41 (1967).
4. R. Lamerton, _Care of the Dying_ (Priority Press Ltd., 1973).
5. Marie Curie Memorial Foundation, "Joint National Cancer Surgery with the Queen's Institute of District Nursing" (Report, 1952).
6. W. D. Rees, "The Distress of Dying," _British Medical Journal_ 3 (1972).
7. R. Lamerton, "Care of the Dying, Pt. IV, The Pains of Death," _Nursing Times_ 69 (January 1973).
8. S. Lack, "I Want to Die While I'm Still Alive," _Death Education_ 1 (1977): 165-76.
9. Saunders, "Terminal Stages of Cancer."
10. Elisabeth Kubler-Ross, _On Death and Dying_ (New York: Macmillan Co., 1969).
11. John Hinton, "Talking with People about to Die," _British Medical Journal_ 3 (1974): 25-27.
12. Lamerton, "Care of the Dying."
13. D. L. Rabin and L. H. Rabin, "Consequences of Death for Physicians, Nurses, and Hospitals," in Brim et al., _The Dying Patient_ (New York: Russell Sage, 1970).
14. R. W. Buckingham, S. A. Lack, et al., "Living with the Dying: Use of the Technique of Participant Observation," _Canadian Medical Association Journal_ 115 (December 18, 1976): 1211-15.
15. Ibid.

16. A. Hackett and M. Weisman, "Reactions to the Imminence of Death," The Threat of Impending Disaster, ed. Grosser (Cambridge: M.I.T. Press, 1964).

17. S. A. Lack, "Philosophy and Organization of a Hospice Program--Psychological Care of the Dying Patient," ed. Charles A. Garfield, University of California School of Medicine (San Francisco, 1977).

18. C. M. Saunders, The Management of Terminal Illness (London: Hospital Medicine Publications, 1967).

19. R. Melzack, The Puzzle of Pain (Harmondsworth, England: Penguin, 1973), p. 142.

20. C. M. Saunders, "The Nursing of Patients Dying of Cancer," Nursing Times 55 (November 6, 1959): 1091-92.

21. Ibid.

22. Ibid.

23. R. G. Twycross, "Clinical Experience with Diamorphine in Advanced Malignant Disease," International Journal of Clinical Pharmacology, Therapy, and Toxicology 9, no. 3 (1974).

24. Ibid.

25. S. A. Lack, "Management of Pain in Terminal Cancer," Medical News-Tribune (England), vol. 4, no. 38, September 18, 1972, 2.

26. B. M. Mount, "Use of the Brompton Mixture in Treating the Chronic Pain of Malignant Disease," Canadian Medical Association Journal 115 (July 17, 1976): 122-24.

27. L. Le Shan, "The World of the Patient in Severe Pain of Long Duration," Journal of Chronic Disease, vol. 17, no. 119 (1974).

28. Mount, "Use of Brompton Mixture."

29. Ibid.

30. Ibid.

31. Melzack, Puzzle of Pain.

32. Mount, "Use of Brompton Mixture."

33. R. Melzack et al., "The Brompton Mixture: Effects on Pain in Cancer Patients," _Canadian Medical Association Journal_ 115 (July 17, 1976): 125-26.

34. Saunders, "The Nursing of Patients Dying."

35. Kubler-Ross, _On Death and Dying._

36. John Hinton, "The Physical and Mental Distress of the Dying," _Quarterly Journal of of Medicine_ 32 (1963) 1.

37. C. M. Parkes, "The Emotional Impact of Cancer on Patients and Their Families," _Journal of Laryngology and Otology_, vol. 89, no. 12 (December 1975), pp. 1271-79.

38. Hinton, "Physical and Mental Distress."

39. Parkes, "Emotional Impact."

40. Ibid., p. 1275.

41. Hinton, "Physical and Mental Distress."

42. Robert L. Williams and Spurgeon Cole, "Religiosity, General Anxiety, and Apprehension Concerning Death," _Journal of Social Psychology_ 75 (1968): 111-17.

43. Hinton, "Physical and Mental Distress."

44. Kubler-Ross, _On Death and Dying._

45. Ibid., pp. 82-85.

46. Ibid., pp. 85-112.

47. J. V. Porter, "A Therapeutic Community for the Dying," _Association of Operating Room Nurses Journal_, vol. 21, no. 5 (April 1975), pp. 838-43.

48. R. J. Carey, "Living Until Death," _Hospital Progress_, vol. 55, no. 2 (February 1974), pp. 82-87.

49. Sigmund B. Kahn and Vincent Zarro, "The Management of the Dying Patient," _Seminars in Drug Treatment_, vol. 3, no. 1 (Summer 1973), pp. 37-45.

50. Arnold J. Rosin, Marcel Assael, and Leah Wallach, "The Influence of Emotional Reaction on the Course of Fatal Illness," _Geriatrics_ (July 1976), pp. 87-90.

51. Parkes, "Emotional Impact."

52. David A. Shephard, "Terminal Care: Towards an Ideal," <u>Canadian Medical Association Journal</u> 115 (July 1976): 97-98.

53. Kubler-Ross, <u>On Death and Dying</u>, p. 9.

54. David Lester et al., "Attitudes of Nursing Students and Nursing Faculty Toward Death," <u>Nursing Research</u>, vol. 23, no. 1 (1974).

55. H. Feifel, "Perception of Death," <u>Annals of the New York Academy of Science</u> 164 (1969): 669.

56. Rosalee Yeaworth et al., "Attitudes of Nursing Students Toward the Dying Patient," <u>Nursing Research</u>, vol. 23, no. 1 (1974), pp. 20-24.

57. R. Lamerton, "Teamwork," <u>Nursing Times</u> (December 1972), pp. 1642-43.

58. Kenneth Davis, "Ergos, Thanatos: The Not-So-Benign Neglect, or Sexuality, Death and the Physician," <u>Texas Reports on Biology and Medicine</u>, vol. 32, no. 1 (Spring 1974), pp. 43-48.

59. B. M. Mount, "The Problem of Caring for the Dying in a General Hospital; The Palliative Care Unit as a Possible Solution," <u>Canadian Medical Association Journal</u> 115 (July 17, 1976), pp. 119-21.

60. C. M. Worby and R. Babineau, "The Family Interview: Helping Patient and Family Cope with Metastatic Disease," <u>Geriatrics</u> (June 1974), pp. 83-94.

61. Lack, "Philosophy and Organization of a Hospice Program."

62. Worby and Babineau, "Family Interview," p. 83.

63. Parkes, "Emotional Impact," p. 1274.

64. Dixie Crase and Darrell Crase, "Live Issues Surrounding Death Education," <u>Journal of School of Health</u> (February 1974), pp. 70-73.

65. R. M. Holford, "Terminal Care," <u>Nursing Times</u> (January 1973), pp. 113-15.

66. W. Dewi Rees and Sylvia G. Lutkins, "Mortality of Bereavement," *British Medical Journal* (October 1967).

67. Mary Ann Rose, "Problems Families Face in Home Care," *American Journal of Nursing* (March 1976), pp. 416-18.

68. Ibid.

69. I. O. Glick, R. S. Weiss, and C. M. Parkes, *The First Year of Bereavement* (New York: J. Wiley and Sons, 1974).

70. Irwin Gerber et al., "Anticipatory Grief and Aged Widows and Widowers," *Journal of Gerontology*, vol. 30, no. 2 (1975), pp. 225-29.

71. John Hinton, "Physical and Mental Distress."

72. Geoffrey Gorer, *Death, Grief and Mourning in Contemporary Britain* (London: Crosset, 1965).

73. R. W. Buckingham et al., "Living with the Dying," p. 1211.

74. Melvin J. Krant and Lee C. Johnston, "An Evaluation of Existential Dimensions of Late-Stage Cancer Patients and their Families," Report from the Tufts Cancer Psychosocial Study Unit (Boston).

CHAPTER 10

Objectives and Methodology of the Study

Editor's Note: The material in this section of
the report is a portion of Robert W.
Buckingham's dissertation.   The reader
interested in more detail on the statistical
methods used in the study is advised to see the
entire dissertation, presented to the Faculty
of the Yale School of Medicine in Candidacy for
the Degree of Doctor of Public Health.

OBJECTIVES OF RESEARCH

The overall goal of this research project
was to evaluate the Hospice Home Care Program
and to determine whether the Hospice staff have
met the stated goal of decreasing the anxiety
and depression experienced by patients and their
primary care persons. Because the quality and
intensity of perceived anxiety and depression
are determined by both physical and psychological processes, the Hospice approach
encompasses treatment of many contributors to
negative affect. The question was whether the
Hospice program of terminal care, by providing
for many needs that often cannot be met in
acute-care settings, is more successful at
relieving these symptoms than are other
facilities for the terminally ill.

METHODOLOGY

Organization of the Study

Design. To establish the effect of Hospice
services, a group that had been part of the
Hospice Home Care Program was compared with a
group that had not, over the study period of
September 1, 1976, to May 31, 1977. The
equivalent group posttest design was employed to
establish the effect of the Home Care Program by
facilitating a comparison of outcomes.[1] This
design is suited to an evaluation of a terminal
care facility in which random assignment was
impossible, subjects were few in number, and
there was insufficient time for a pretest.

To find evidence for or against the thesis
that the Hospice Home Care Program provides
effective care to its terminal patients, a
comparison was made between the anxiety,
depression, and social adjustment scores of the
Hospice and non-Hospice patient-family groups.
These two groups were measured using three
self-report questionnaires--the Symptom
Checklist,[2] Social Adjustment Self-report,[3]
and Zuckerman and Lubin Adjective Checklist.[4]

The self-report mode of psychological
measurement was selected because it provides
access to information that is unobtainable
through other channels. Responses are those of
the subject, not of an objective clinical
observer whose report, however insightful, is
based only on verbal and behavioral manifestations of affect. Although question bias may be
undetected, self-report instruments eliminate
interviewer bias; they can also economize
administrative and scoring time. Moreover, if
a trained representative monitors the completion
of the questionnaire, complete data can usually
be obtained.

<u>Hypotheses</u>. The following hypotheses were tested:

1. Hospice patients will exhibit lower levels of anxiety and depression as measured by the Zuckerman Adjective Checklist and the Symptom Checklist-90 scales than will the patients in the non-Hospice comparison group.
2. Hospice patients will exhibit higher levels of social adjustment as measured by the Social Adjustment Self-Report Questionnaire than will the patients in the non-Hospice comparison group.
3. Hospice primary care persons will exhibit lower levels of anxiety and depression as measured by the Zuckerman Adjective Checklist and the Symptom Checklist than will primary care persons in the non-Hospice comparison group.
4. Hospice primary care persons will exhibit higher levels of social adjustment as measured by the Social Adjustment Self-Report Questionnaire than will primary care persons in the comparison non-Hospice group.

<u>Sample</u> <u>selection</u>. All patients in the Hospice program enter during the terminal stages of cancer, with a clinical prognosis of six months or less. More than 50 percent of this total population have cancer with a primary site of lung, colon, or breast. The questionnaire was administered to patients who survived the program more than two weeks and who had a projected survival time of three months or less. In total, 39 patients made up the Hospice sample. The three designated primary sites were specified as criteria for admittance into the study to facilitate the acquisition of a matched control group. The comparative sample consisted

213

of patients who met all criteria for acceptance into the Hospice program except that they did not reside within the Hospice geographical service area.

In summary, members of both groups had a confirmed diagnosis of terminal cancer with a projected survival time of three months or less; lived with a friend or relative who could function as a primary care person; were no younger than 18; and had been referred by the same oncologists as had referred the Hospice population in general.

The total number of patients comprising the control sample was 35. These patients were matched with the Hospice group with respect to age (within 10 years), sex, and primary site of cancer.

Background Data

Demographic and Medical information. For Hospice patients, demographic data regarding age, sex, education, occupation, and financial circumstances were obtained from existing records, from items in the self-report questionnaire, and from the Hospice routine data retrieval system. Information concerning ethnic background, religion, and religiosity was gathered in the same manner. Similar demographic and cultural data were compiled for Hospice primary care persons. The relationship of the primary care person to the patient was also noted. The history of the patient's terminal illness, prognosis, major medical complications, and awareness of illness were obtained through the data retrieval system.

For the control group patients and their primary care persons, demographic data regarding age, sex, education, occupation, and financial circumstances, as well as information concerning ethnic background, religion, and religiosity were obtained from questionnaire items, routine forms, and records kept by the primary physician. This information, along with the history of the patient's terminal illness, was extracted from the medical records with the consent of the primary physician.

Research Instruments

Symptom Checklist-90. The SCL-90 is a 90-item, self-report symptom inventory developed by the Clinical Psychometrics Research unit of Johns Hopkins University. It was designed to reflect the nature of psychological symptoms experienced by psychiatric and medical patients.[5] The instrument serves as a measure of current, point-in-time, psychological symptom status. Although it is not a measure of personality, certain personality types or disorders may exhibit a characteristic profile of primary symptoms.

Each item of the SCL-90 is rated on a five-point scale of distress, with a choice of responses ranging from "not at all" at the lowest pole to "extremely" at the highest. Scoring and interpretation are in terms of nine primary symptom dimensions:

1. somatization (distress arising from perceptions of bodily dysfunction; cardiovascular, gastrointestinal and respiratory complaints; headaches, pain and discomfort of the gross muscula-ture, etc.),

2. obsessive-compulsive (thoughts, impulses, and actions experienced as persistent and irresistible by the individual, yet of an ego-alien nature),

3. interpersonal sensitivity (feelings of

215

personal inferiority and inadequacy in comparison to others; self-deprecation and feelings of discomfort and uneasiness with others),

4. depression (withdrawal of life interest, diminished motivation, loss of vital energy, and dysphoric affect and mood; cognitive and somatic correlates of depression such as hopelessness and suicidal thoughts),

5. anxiety (general signs of anxiety such as nervousness, tension, trembling, and panic attacks; cognitive components involving feelings of apprehension, terror, and dread; certain somatic indications),

6. hostility (aggression, rage, irritability, and resentment; symptoms of anger in the form of thoughts, feelings, or actions),

7. phobic anxiety (persistent, irrational, and disproportionate fear and avoidance response to a specific person, place, object, or situation),

8. paranoid ideation (paranoid behavior as a consequence of a disordered mode of thinking),

9. and psychoticism (a graduated continuum of measurement sensitive to a range of psychoticism from interpersonal alienation to dramatic psychosis).

Three global indices have also been developed from the items of the instrument, each of which reflects a distinct aspect of the patient's general psychological state.

1. The Global Severity Index (GSI) represents the best single indicator of the current level of the disorder and is designed for use in instances where a summary measure is required.

2. The Positive Symptom Distress Index (PSDI) measures response style: whether the patient is "augmenting" or "attenuating" symptomatic distress in his style of reporting his disorder.
3. The Positive Symptom Total (PST) is a simple count of the number of symptoms the patient experiences to any degree.

Zuckerman Adjective Checklist. The Zuckerman and Lubin Adjective Checklist was developed as a self-report instrument capable of measuring transient depressive mood, feeling, or emotion, as opposed to more chronic, enduring depressive states.[6] Economy and ease of administration, high face validity, and indications of ready acceptance by subjects were all considerations favoring the selection of this instrument. The list consisted of 27 words descriptive of affect and aspects of personality functioning that subjects identified as related or unrelated to their present feelings.

Social Adjustment Self-Report. The Social Adjustment Self-Report (SAS-SR) was designed to measure social adjustment by gathering information about the patient's interpersonal or expressive role performance in six major areas of functioning: work as a housewife, student, or worker; social and leisure activities, relationships with extended family; and roles as a spouse, parent, and member of a family unit.[7] The questions in each of these areas fall into four main categories: performance at expected tasks, degree of friction with others, finer aspects of interpersonal relations, and inner feelings and satisfaction. Each question is rated on a five-point scale with a higher score indicating maladjustment.

217

Reliability and Validity of Questionnaires

The reliability of an instrument or method of quality assessment is the degree to which results are reproducible when the assessment is repeated. The reliability of the SCL-90 symptom dimensions has been determined by Derogatis and others in terms of two measures: internal consistency and test-retest. The former measures the homogeneity or consistency with which the items representing each symptom construct mirror the underlying factor. Satisfactory consistency was found.[8] Test-retest reliability, an indicator of stability of measurement across time, was measured by Derogatis on the SCL-90 in terms of coefficients obtained from a sample of 94 heterogeneous psychiatric outpatients, and was found to reach an appropriate level for measures of symptom constructs.[9]

Lubin administered the Zuckerman Checklist together with 13 similar depression adjective checklists to a group of 48 male and 78 female subjects.[10] In his subsequent examination of the correlations among the 14 lists he separated the lists into two sets. Within each set the lists were treated as alternate forms since none contained overlapping adjectives. The interlist correlations were considered as alternate form reliabilities: In all cases the correlations were significant at well below the 0.001 level. High intercorrelation had been previously demonstrated by Lubin[11] and was perceived as a possible indication of equivalence among the adjective checklists tested.

Validity refers to whether a test measures what it purports to measure. At the operational level, validation consists of a set of correlational procedures by which the scale to be validated is correlated with inclusive measures of the construct which the scale attempts to represent. Some important aspects of validity have been documented for the SCL-90 despite its recent origins.[12]

Evidence for validity of the Zuckerman Adjective Checklist has been presented by Lubin, who compared the Zuckerman list with six other depression adjective checklists in a cross-validation study using an analysis of variance techniques.[13] Correlations between seven lists and two additional measures of depression, the Minnesota Multiphasic Personality Inventory-Depression (MMPI--D) Scale[14] and the Beck Inventory of Depression[15] were also calculated. All correlations were found to be significant at least at the 0.005 level. Lubin elicited similar results in subsequent analyses yielding significant alternate form reliability and concurrent validity data.[16]

Validity of the Social Adjustment Self-Report has been claimed on the basis of comparison to data from the interview form from which it was derived. Correlations between the interview and the self-report were found to be significant.[17]

Reliability of Sample Data

An estimate of reliability based on the average correlation among items within a test is said to concern the "internal consistency." The size of the reliability coefficient is actually based on both the average correlation among items (the internal consistency) and the number of items.[18] The internal consistency reliability was determined by means of coefficient alpha[19] for the scores of the Symptom Checklist 90 and Social Adjustment Adjective Self-Report. The special version of alpha applicable to dichotomous items (Kuder

Estimates of Reliability for Psychosocial Scores of
Hospice and Non-Hospice Patients and Primary Care Persons
New Haven, 1977

	Number of items	Patients Hospice & Non-Hospice pooled N = 74	Primary Care Persons Hospice & Non-Hospice pooled N = 74
Kuder-Richardson Formula 20			
From Zuckerman			
Anxiety	10	.99	.95
Depression	9	.99	.97
Hostility	8	.99	.96
Coefficient alpha			
From SCL-90			
Somatization	12	.96	.93
Interpersonal sensitivity	9	.97	.89
Depression	13	.96	.90
Anxiety	10	.97	.91
Hostility	6	.96	.86

(continued)

Estimates of Reliability (continued)

From SAS-SR			
Mean social adjustment score	8	.75	.46
Work outside the home	6	.94	.98
Work at home as a housewife	6	.97	.98
Social & leisure activities	12	.91	.80
Relationship with extended family	8	.96	.89
Relationship with spouse	9	.97	.96
Fulfillment of parental role	4	.98	.99
Functioning within family unit	3	.90	.82
Performance at work	4	.96	.96
Friction	8	.80	.58
Inhibited communication	7	.76	.61
Submissive-dependent	3	.77	.63
Family attachment	3	.46	.31
Anxious rumination	7	.74	.66

Richardson Formula 20) was used to determine this reliability of the Zuckerman Adjective Checklist scores. The reliability coefficients obtained for each of the multiple-item indexes of the tests employed in the study are listed on the following pages. All coefficients were greater than 0.50, except those pertaining to family attachment and mean social adjustment of primary care persons.

Questionnaire Administration and Scoring

The SCL-90, the Social Adjustment Self-Report, and the Zuckerman Adjective Checklist were administered to the Hospice patient and his or her primary care person under the guidance of the Director of Research and Evaluation in a single home visit occurring after two weeks of Hospice Home Care service had been experienced. Members of the control group were interviewed in a similar manner.

The SCL-90 typically required 15 to 20 minutes of the approximately 45-minute interview period to complete, although administration time varied with the circumstances of the interview. The last seven days in a respondent's time frame was designated as the period of recall in answering the questions on the SCL-90 in order to obtain the most relevant information regarding current clinical status.

The Zuckerman Adjective Checklist was completed by the patient and the primary care person as a self-report under the guidance of the Director of Research and Evaluation. The subject was directed to respond to the items in the checklist according to his mood and feelings on the day of the interview. A scoring key consisted of differentiating adjectives which separate depressed from nondepressed subjects. The average length of time required by the patients to complete the Zuckerman Adjective Checklist was approximately three minutes, a distinct advantage with very sick patients who tire easlly.

The SAS-SR, a self-report questionnaire, was completed by both the patient and the primary care person under the direction of the Director of Research and Evaluation. The SAS-SR questionnaire assesses the patient's functioning during the preceding two-week period. The instrument was designed to be analyzed by inspection of an <u>overall</u> <u>adjustment</u> <u>score</u> which is a sum of all items over the number of scored items, and a <u>role</u> <u>area</u> <u>mean</u> <u>score</u>, obtained by totaling the scores of all items in a role area and dividing by the sum of items actually scored in that area.

The Social Adjustment Self-Report measured very specific aspects of social adjustment. Therefore, not all of the items were pertinent for all subjects. For example, performance at work could be measured only for those individuals who were indeed working (and most patients and many primary care persons were not).

In all cases, composite scores were assigned proportionately on the basis of the answers that a respondent did give. For example, assume that six items were combined in a single dimension score with scores of 1, 2, 3, 4, or 5 assigned to each item, as in the SCL-90 instruments. The respondent could achieve a maximum score of $\frac{30}{6}$ or 5. If a given respondent answered only five of the items but received a score of five on those items, he would be given a proportionate score of $\frac{25}{5} = 5$ on the index. The respondent who received a score of 3 on the four items answered would be given a final score of $\frac{12}{4} = 3$. When these computations resulted in fractional results, rounding off was employed to simplify the final index scores. Composite scores were also assigned proportionately for the Zuckerman Checklist, in which scores of 0 or 1 were assigned to each item.

DATA ANALYSIS

Statistical Tests

The principal objectives of the study were
to determine whether Hospice patients and primary care persons exhibit lower levels of
anxiety and depression as measured by the
Zuckerman Checklist and Symptom Checklist 90
instruments, and higher levels of social
adjustment as measured by the Social Adjustment
Self-Report instrument than do non-Hospice
patients and primary care persons. To carry out
these objectives, the data were first examined
to determine the nature of the statistical
comparisons that could be performed. The
choice of the statistical tests to be used in
the comparison of mean values of variables
measuring anxiety, depression, and social
adjustment was contingent upon the assumptions
regarding the distribution of the Hospice and
non-Hospice groups.

Nonparametric analysis. The sign test was
used in attempting to detect differences between
the Hospice and control groups on psychosocial
scores. The data, which were matched with
respect to the relevant extraneous variables,
age, sex, and primary disease site, were found
to be suitable for use of the sign test, which
makes no assumptions regarding the form of the
distribution of differences, but assumes
independence between variables. The null
hypothesis tested by the sign test is that:

$$p(X_{Hospice} > X_{non-Hospice}) = p(X_{Hospice} < X_{non-Hospice})$$

where $X_{Hospice}$ and $X_{non-Hospice}$ are the

two scores for a matched pair consisting of a Hospice patient and a non-Hospice patient of the same age, sex, and primary disease site.

The difference between the scores of every Hospice and non-Hospice member of a matched pair was inspected and recorded as either plus or minus. According to the null hypothesis, positive and negative values of that difference are equally likely. The probability associated with the occurrence of a particular number of pluses and minuses was determined by reference to the binomial distribution with P = Q, where N = number of pairs. If a matched pair showed no difference, it was dropped from the analysis and N was thereby reduced. The null hypothesis was rejected if too few differences of one sign occurred.[20]

Analysis based on the assumption of a normal distribution. Because of the potentially useful insights that may be gained, it was decided to make use of the independent t-test and the paired t-test and to relax the requirement of a probability sample. Although the requirements for such an analysis may not be fully met by the data, t-tests may help in judging whether differences between the Hospice and control groups regarding important variable are significant. Paired t-tests were used to compare mean psychosocial scores of matched pairs, and independent t-tests were used to compare mean group scores.

Limitations of the Study

Sample. Before summarizing the findings of this project, it is necessary to insert a word of caution regarding interpretation of the data. The study represents an attempt to explore

226

certain psychosocial parameters for a limited subset of the Hospice patient and primary care person population--namely, for all breast, lung, and colon cancer patients and their primary care persons. Because the study aims at evaluating Hospice Home Care services, one of its implicit goals is to apply its findings to other subsets of the Hospice population. However, such generalizations are limited. It was hoped that the patients and primary care persons included in the study were representative of Hospice, New Haven, patients and primary care persons in general. But because cancer of some primary sites is more painful than cancer of other sites and is characterized by different symptoms and degrees of disfigurement, the study sample may not be representative.

The ethical, political, and practical situation in which the study was carried out also placed certain limitations on the volume and characteristics of the data. The small size and diversity of the Hospice population precluded the selection of a random sample; indeed, the sample obtained by taking all eligible patients in the study period was still quite small. The possibility exists that differences between the groups on variables of interest came about through the differential recruitment of persons making up the groups. The groups might have differed on levels of anxiety, depression, and social adjustment even without Hospice services. However, to avoid excluding potential recipients of Hospice care from the Hospice Home Care Program, the non-Hospice sample came from outside the Hospice geographical service area and thus could not be said to have selectively avoided exposure to Hospice service.

Dropouts. Another possible source of differences between the groups might have been

the differential dropout of persons. Of the
original number of patients, 11 percent of those
in the control group sample and 10 percent of
those in the Hospice sample were unable to
respond due to weakness and incoherence.
However, the excluded patients were not different from the rest of the sample on other
relevant characteristics (for example, ethnic
background and financial status).

Demographic differences. Differences
between the groups in demographic characteristics that might influence psychosocial scores
are a potential source of bias. Documentation
that the Hospice and control groups are similar
on variables relevant to the comparison is basic
to the final comparison of outcomes. Because
the study groups were matched on diagnosis,
estimated prognosis, primary site of cancer,
and, as closely as possible, on age, it was
expected that the groups would be similar. (See
Tables 57-70.) They were nearly equivalent on
the distribution of primary site of the disease,
sex, age of patient, race, marital status, and
religion.

However, there were differences between
the Hospice and control groups which seemed to
be related to the area from which they came.
For example, whereas 30 percent of patients and
primary care persons in the Hospice group were
of Italian extraction, only 10 percent of
patients and primary care persons in the
control group were. Similarly, although the
mean educational level was the same for the
Hospice and non-Hospice primary care persons,
the distribution of educational levels seemed
to differ between the two primary care person
groups. The two groups were similar with
regard to the occupation of the primary care
persons.

228

Thus, the selection of a control group from outside the Hospice geographical service area apparently led to the introduction of potentially confounding demographic differences between the study groups. Ethnic variations could possibly account for differences in the social adjustment and style of response of patients from the different study groups. Discrepancies in the distribution of educational and occupational levels between the two groups might cause differences in the scores on psychosocial valuables of interest.[21]

In addition, the stresses of terminal illness for the primary care person might vary as a function of age. This might produce differences in the response of the two groups of primary care persons. The Hospice group had primary care persons who were apparently older than the primary care persons in the non-Hospice group.

It is thus evident that any comparative analysis of psychosocial scores between the two study groups must take into account extraneous differences between them or demonstrate that such differences are not significant.

Other potential sources of bias. As is the case with any study attempting to evaluate a federally funded service program, the gratitude of patients and primary care persons receiving free care and their unwillingness to seem critical of such care are potential sources of study bias. The introduction of fee-for-services Hospices with comparable evaluation programs might determine whether this bias was present.

It was the observation of the researcher that patient responses were not influenced by the effects of medication. However, approximately 30 percent of the patient visits were cancelled because the patient's disease had progressed to a stage in which they were too fatigued or incoherent and confused to respond. As the number of people encountered in such a condition was similar across groups, the situation was not considered to be an important source of study bias.

Research Problems

Great problems in sampling arose as a result of the study criterion of an estimated three month prognosis. Although the Hospice admission policy specifically designates a prognosis of six months or less, few Hospice patients survived three months on the program. The mean length of program stay for Hospice patients to date has been 2.2 months. Many patients who otherwise would have qualified for the study died before an adequate amount of time with Hospice care had elapsed to conclude that Hospice was really an intervention. In contrast, non-Hospice patients usually outlived their prognosis and lasted three months or longer. As a consequence, non-Hospice patients were, on the average, more astute and less weak than Hospice patients while being tested. The fact that Hospice patients were more terminal than non-Hospice patients derived from difficulty in making a clinical prognosis, and must, therefore, be considered a current problem inherent in such research involving the terminally ill.

The practical problems of obtaining a sample of patients and family members to interview cannot be overestimated. A major problem in the Hospice group was getting approval through the nurses for a research visit to take place. The nurses did not feel it was their clinical duty to make arrangements for research

activities and often felt obligated to protect
their patients from the inconvenience of what
they saw as intrusions. In addition, patients
were often too weak to be interviewed by the
time they qualified for the study.

Problems of a different nature arose while
attempting to organize a control group sample.
With the assistance of Dr. James Collins, a
clinical professor of therapeutic radiology at
Yale School of Medicine, and the cooperation of
Uncas on Thames Hospital, a control group was
obtained. Fortunately, a greater number of
patients qualified by primary disease site in
the non-Hospice than in the Hospice group. However, much difficulty was experienced in getting
a prognosis of three months or less. Non-
Hospice physicians were less likely to commit
themselves to a specific prognosis than Hospice
physicians; the three-month estimate was usually
a clinical judgment made by a member of the
nursing staff.

Although the Social Adjustment Self-Report
Questionnaire was selected because it is a
sensitive measure of specific aspects of social
adjustment, its format and coding scheme were a
source of confusion to many subjects. Ambiguous
answers resulted when subjects responded to
questions which were not clearly categorized as
applicable to them. Slight revisions in the
questionnaire would alleviate this problem. The
Zuckerman Checklist, although not as sensitive a
measure as the Social Adjustment Self-Report or
the Symptom Checklist-90 instruments, proved to
be an excellent instrument for use with terminal
patients due to its content and brevity. Of the
three questionnaires, the Symptom Checklist-90
is most highly recommended for studies of this
nature. It was readily understood and brief,
and it generated relevant, reliable data.

TABLE 57

Study Group:
Age of Patients

Age in years	Total	Hospice	Non-Hospice
Total Number	(73)	(38)	(35)
Total Percentage	99.9	100.1	100.0
36-50	12.3	13.2	11.4
51-60	19.2	18.4	20.0
61-63	16.4	13.2	20.0
64-66	16.4	18.4	14.3
67-69	16.4	13.2	20.0
70-83	19.2	23.7	14.3
Mean		63.32	62.86
Standard Deviation		10.32	8.11

Significance of T Statistic (2-Tailed
  Probability) > 0.50.

NOTES:
  Percentages do not total 100.0% due to rounding.
  The table excludes one person for whom age was
not ascertained.

TABLE 58

Study Group:
Sex of Patients

Sex	Total	Hospice	Non-Hospice
Total Number	(73)	(38)	(35)
Total Percentage	100.0	100.0	100.0
Male	31.5	28.9	34.3
Female	68.5	71.1	65.7

Chi square = 1.15   with 1 degree of freedom
significance > 0.10

NOTE: The table excludes one person for whom
sex was not ascertained.

TABLE 59

Study Group:
Primary Disease Site

Primary Site	Total	Hospice	Non-Hospice
Total Number	(73)	(38)	(35)
Total Percentage	100.0	100.0	100.1
Breast	35.6	28.9	42.9
Colon	41.1	47.4	34.3
Lung	23.3	23.7	22.9

Chi square = 2.67   with 2 degrees of freedom
significance > 0.10

NOTES:
  Percentages do not total 100.0% due to rounding.
  The table excludes one person for whom primary site was not ascertained.

234

TABLE 60

Study Group: Primary Disease Site by Sex of Patients

Primary Site of Cancer	Total		Hospice		Non-Hospice	
	Male	Female	Male	Female	Male	Female
Total Number	(23)	(49)	(11)	(26)	(12)	(23)
Total Percentage	100.0	100.0	100.0	100.0	100.0	100.0
Breast	--	53.1	--	42.3	--	65.2
Colon	60.9	30.6	72.7	34.6	50.0	26.1
Lung	39.1	16.3	27.3	23.1	50.0	8.7

NOTE: The table excludes one person for whom primary disease site was not ascertained.

TABLE 61

Study Group:
Marital Status of Patients

Marital Status	Total	Hospice	Non-Hospice
Total Number	(73)	(38)	(35)
Total Percentage	99.9	100.1	99.9
Single/Divorced/ Separated	12.3	13.2	11.4
Married	71.2	71.1	71.4
Widowed	16.4	15.8	17.1

Chi square = 1.87 with 2 degrees of freedom
significance > 0.50

NOTES:
  Percentages do not total 100.0% due to
rounding.
  The table excludes one person for whom marital
status was not ascertained.

236

TABLE 62

Study Group:
Race of Patients

Race	Total	Hospice	Non-Hospice
Total Number	(73)	(38)	(35)
Total Percentage	100.0	100.0	100.0
White	93.2	94.7	91.4
Black/Hispanic	6.8	5.3	8.6

Chi square = 0.01   with 1 degree of freedom
significance > 0.50

NOTE: The table excludes one person for whom race was not ascertained.

TABLE 63

Study Group:
Ethnic Background of Patients

Ethnic Background	Total	Hospice	Non-Hospice
Total Number	(73)	(38)	(35)
Total Percentage	100.0	100.0	99.9
Italian	23.3	34.2	11.4
Irish	12.3	15.8	8.6
Anglo-Saxon/British	17.8	18.4	17.1
German/Scandinavian	17.8	18.4	17.1
Other	28.8	13.2	45.7

Chi square = 12.50 with 4 degrees of freedom
significance < 0.05

NOTES:

Percentages do not total 100.0% due to rounding.

The table excludes one person for whom ethnic background was not ascertained.

*Includes Russian-Polish, Puerto-Rican, Afro-American, and combination.

TABLE 64

Study Group:
Religion of Patients

Religion	Total	Hospice	Non-Hospice
Total Number	(70)	(36)	(34)
Total Percentage	100.0	100.0	100.0
Protestant	35.7	27.8	44.1
Catholic	64.3	72.2	55.9

Chi square = 2.04   with 1 degree of freedom
significance > 0.10

NOTE: The table excludes those persons (4.1% of total) who reported being Jewish or having no religion, and one person whose religion was not ascertained.

TABLE 65

Study Group:
Educational Level of Patients

Educational Level	Total	Hospice	Non-Hospice
Total Number	(73)	(38)	(35)
Total Percentage	99.9	100.0	100.0
Partial college, business college, or stand. univ. training	16.4	23.7	28.6
High school graduate	43.8	36.8	31.4
Partial high school or less training	39.7	39.5	40.0

Chi square = 4.33   with 2 degrees of freedom
significance > 0.10

NOTES:

Percentages do not total 100.0% due to rounding.

The table excludes one person for whom education was not ascertained.

TABLE 66

Study Group: Occupation of Patients

Occupation	Total	Hospice	Non-Hospice
Total Number	(71)	(36)	(35)
Total Percentage	100.0	100.0	100.0
Business manager, proprietor of medium-size business (35,000-100,000), lesser professional or graduate student, administrative personnel, small independent business (6,000-35,000)	19.7	16.7	22.8
Clerical and sales worker, technician or owner of little business or undergraduate student	38.0	38.9	37.1
Skilled manual employee	26.8	25.0	28.6
Machine operator, semi-skilled employee, unskilled employee, unemployed—no previous job skill	15.5	19.4	11.5

Chi square = 1.17   with 3 degrees of freedom   significance > 0.10

NOTES:
  The table excludes those persons (4.05% of total) for whom occupation was not ascertained.
  If patient was housewife, husband's profession was recorded.

241

TABLE 67

Study Group:
Financial Status of Patients

Financial Status	Total	Hospice	Non-Hospice
Total Number	(70)	(35)	(35)
Total Percentage	100.0	99.9	100.1
Less than $5,000	50.0	37.1	62.9
$5,000-$7,000	24.3	25.7	22.9
$7,000-$15,000	25.7	37.1	14.3

Significance of T Statistic (2-Tailed
probability) < 0.01.

NOTES:
   Percentages do not total 100.0 due to rounding.
   The table excludes those persons (5.41% of
total) for whom financial status was not ascertained.

TABLE 68

Study Group:
Hollingshead Score of Patients

Hollingshead Score	Total	Hospice	Non-Hospice
Total Number	(73)	(38)	(35)
Total Percentage	100.0	100.0	100.0
I, II, or III	27.4	34.2	20.0
IV	57.5	47.4	68.6
V	15.1	18.4	11.4

Significance of T Statistic (2-Tailed probability) > 0.10.

NOTES:

The table excludes one person for whom Hollingshead Score was not ascertained.

On the Hollingshead scale the numeral I represents the highest social class (in terms of occupation and education) and V represents the lowest.

TABLE 69

Study Group: Demographic Characteristics
of Primary Care Persons

| | Primary Care Persons | |
	Hospice	Non-Hospice
Total Number	39	35
Total Percentage	100.0	100.0
Sex		
Male	38.5	20.0
Female	59.0	80.0
N.A.	2.6	--
Age		
18-45	33.3	45.7
46-55	12.8	31.4
56-60	20.5	14.3
61-65	20.5	2.9
66-75	2.6	2.9
76 and over	5.1	2.9
N.A.	5.1	2.9
Mean Age	51.3	46.5
Race		
White	92.3	91.4
Black	5.1	5.7
Hispanic	--	2.9
N.A.	2.6	--
Marital Status		
Single (never married)	5.1	2.9
Married	89.7	85.7
Divorced/Widowed/ Separated	2.6	11.4
N.A.	2.6	--

(continued)

TABLE 69 (cont.)

| | Primary Care Persons | |
	Hospice	Non-Hospice
Ethnic Background		
Italian	33.3	14.3
Irish	12.8	2.9
Anglo-Saxon British	5.1	14.3
German/Scandinavian	7.7	11.4
Other	41.0	57.2
Occupation		
1 Higher executive or business manager	10.3	2.9
2 Small independent business	20.5	31.4
3 Clerical-sales worker	28.2	34.3
4 Skilled manual employee	15.4	22.9
5 Semi-skilled/ unskilled/unemployed	20.5	5.7
N.A.	5.1	2.9
Education		
Graduate or professional training	2.6	2.9
College graduate	5.1	
Business college	20.5	25.7
High school graduate	30.8	65.7
Partial high school	12.8	5.7
Completed grades 7-9	20.5	--
Less than 7 years	5.1	--
N.A.	2.6	--
Religion		
Protestant	28.9	42.9
Catholic	68.4	57.1
Jewish/No Religion	2.6	--

(continued)

TABLE 69 (cont.)

	Primary Care Persons	
	Hospice	Non-Hospice
Practicing Religion		
Yes	51.3	42.9
No	46.2	57.1
N.A.	2.6	--
Financial Information		
Less than $5,000	23.1	11.4
$5,000-7,000	15.4	25.7
$7,000-9,000	5.1	17.1
$9,000-11,000	17.9	28.6
$11,000-13,000	10.3	11.4
$13,000-15,000	12.8	2.9
$15,000+	12.8	2.9
N.A.	2.6	--
Hollingshead Score		
I	2.6	2.9
II	12.8	2.9
III	23.1	40.0
IV	43.6	51.4
V	15.4	2.9
N.A.	--	--
Mean	3.487	3.486

NOTES:

Percentages may not total 100.0% due to rounding.

N.A.= Not ascertained

On the Hollingshead scale the numeral I represents the highest social class (in terms of occupation and education) and V represents the lowest.

TABLE 70

Study Group: Demographic Characteristics of Patients
by Primary Disease Site

	Hospice			Non-Hospice		
	Breast	Colon	Lung	Breast	Colon	Lung
Number	12	18	9	15	12	8
Mean Age	66.50	62.35	60.89	60.87	63.50	65.63
	%	%	%	%	%	%
Sex						
Male	--	50.0	33.3	--	50.0	75.0
Female	100.0	50.0	66.7	100.0	50.0	25.0
Race						
White	100.0	94.4	77.7	100.0	83.3	87.5
Black	--	--	22.3	--	8.3	12.5
Hispanic	--	5.6	--	--	8.3	--
Marital Status						
Single	8.3	16.6	--	--	8.3	25.0
Married	50.0	72.2	88.9	73.3	66.7	75.0
Divorced	--	5.6	--	6.7	--	--
Widowed	33.3	5.6	11.1	20.0	25.0	--
Separated	8.3	--	--	--	--	--

(continued)

248

Table 70 - continued

Ethnic Background

Italian	25.0	38.9	33.3	13.3	16.7	--
Russian-Polish	8.3	--	--	6.7	--	12.5
Irish	33.3	5.6	11.1	13.3	8.3	--
Puerto Rican	--	--	--	--	8.3	--
Anglo-Saxon/British	16.7	16.7	22.2	13.3	16.7	25.0
German-Scandinavian	16.7	22.2	11.1	13.3	16.7	25.0
Other	--	11.1	--	33.3	8.3	12.5
Combination	--	--	--	6.7	16.7	12.5
Afro-American	--	5.6	22.2	--	8.3	12.5

Education

College graduate	--	--	22.2	--	--	--
Part. college/bus. college	16.7	--	11.1	--	--	37.5
High school graduate	41.6	22.2	22.2	66.7	50.0	25.0
Partial high school	16.7	38.9	11.1	20.0	50.0	25.0
Completed 7-9 grade	8.3	27.8	11.1	6.7	--	--
Less than 7 yrs school	16.7	11.1	22.2	6.7	--	12.5

Religion

Catholic	75.0	72.2	55.6	73.3	41.7	37.5
Protestant	16.7	27.8	33.3	20.0	58.3	62.5
Jew	8.3	--	--	6.7	--	--
No Religion	--	--	11.1	--	--	--

Table 70 - continued

	Hospice			Non-Hospice		
	Breast	Colon	Lung	Breast	Colon	Lung
Number	12	18	9	15	12	8
	%	%	%	%	%	%
Practicing religion						
Yes	66.7	50.0	44.4	53.3	41.7	50.0
No	33.3	50.0	55.6	46.7	58.3	50.0
Occupation						
Business manager/propriet. of mid-size business	8.3	5.6	11.1	--	--	25.0
Small ind. business	16.7	--	11.1	13.3	16.7	25.0
Clerical sales worker	16.7	44.4	44.4	53.3	25.0	25.0
Skilled manual employee	16.7	27.8	22.2	20.0	50.0	12.5
Machine operator/ semi-skilled employee	16.7	16.7	--	6.7	8.3	12.5
Unskilled employee	8.3	--	--	--	--	--
Unemployed--no previous job skill	16.7	5.6	11.1	6.7	--	--

Table 70 - continued

Financial status

Less than $5,000	41.7	44.4	11.1	60.0	58.3	75.0
$5,000–7,000	16.7	22.2	44.5	20.0	25.0	25.0
$7,000–9,000	--	5.6	--	13.3	--	--
$9,000–11,000	16.7	11.1	22.2	--	8.3	--
$11,000–13,000	--	11.1	--	6.7	--	--
$13,000–15,000	25.0	5.6	--	--	8.3	--
$15,000+	--	--	22.2	--	--	--

NOTE: Percentages may not add to 100.0% due to rounding.

TABLE 71

Mean Scores of Psychosocial Variables for
Hospice and Non-Hospice Patients and Primary Care Persons

| Variable | Hospice | | Non-Hospice | |
	Patients	Primary Care Persons	Patients	Primary Care Persons
From Zuckerman*				
Anxiety	.42	.50	.68	.78
Depression	.41	.45	.51	.59
Hostility	.14	.22	.37	.45
From SCL-90**				
Somatization	1.90	1.46	2.46	2.17
Interpersonal sensitivity	1.40	1.48	2.21	2.05
Depression	2.12	1.90	2.91	2.84
Anxiety	1.65	1.60	2.16	2.34
Hostility	1.37	1.60	2.16	2.34

252

(continued)

Table 71 - continued

From SAS-SR***

Mean social adjustment score	2.11	1.86	2.28	2.33
Work outside the home	4.48	2.52	5.00	2.83
Work at home as a housewife	3.08	1.66	2.92	2.62
Social & leisure activities	2.36	2.03	2.66	2.69
Relationship with extended family	1.61	1.57	1.96	2.06
Relationship with spouse	2.18	1.97	2.54	2.42
Fulfillment of parental role	1.48	1.69	1.76	2.23
Functioning within family unit	1.78	1.94	2.44	2.26
Enough money to care for own & family's financial need	1.58	1.76	1.30	1.74
Performance at work	3.74	1.86	3.32	2.90
Friction	1.23	1.47	1.96	2.10
Inhibited communication	2.10	1.84	2.20	2.35
Submissive-dependent	1.61	1.56	2.31	2.21
Family attachment	2.66	2.08	2.94	2.55
Anxious rumination	2.01	1.84	2.35	2.38

*0 = not at all; 1 = extremely
**1 = not at all; 5 = extremely
***1 = functioning well; 5 = extremely maladjusted

253

TABLE 72

Mean Scores of Psychosocial Variables for
Patients Categorized by Primary Disease Site

Variable	Hospice			Non-Hospice		
	Breast	Colon	Lung	Breast	Colon	Lung
N	12	18	9	15	12	8
From Zuckerman*						
Anxiety	.36	.46	.41	.76	.59	.66
Depression	.40	.40	.44	.60	.43	.49
Hostility	.18	.13	.13	.43	.30	.36
From SCI-90**						
Somatization	1.99	1.82	1.92	2.85	2.23	2.66
Interpersonal sensitivity	1.51	1.44	1.18	2.62	1.99	2.42
Depression	2.13	2.17	1.99	2.64	2.39	2.58
Anxiety	1.83	1.63	1.46	2.65	2.18	2.58
Hostility	1.39	1.41	1.27	2.43	1.91	2.31

(continued)

Table 72 - continued
From SAS-SR***

Mean social adjustment score	2.05	2.33	1.71	1.41	1.29	1.07
Work outside the home	--	--	1.33	.18	.15	.15
Work at home as a housewife	3.11	3.24	2.50	2.09	1.07	.94
Social and leisure activities	2.17	2.48	2.42	2.19	1.96	2.05
Relationship w/extended family	1.53	1.74	1.48	1.69	1.87	1.52
Relationship w/spouse	2.39	2.13	2.02	2.42	2.09	2.08
Fulfillment of parental role	1.33	1.46	2.00	.72	.77	.25
Functioning within family unit	1.89	1.97	1.24	1.88	1.86	1.50
Enough money to care for own & family's financial need	1.64	1.80	1.00	1.53	1.83	1.13
Performance at work	3.81	3.19	3.17	1.85	.88	.88
Friction	1.37	1.15	1.15	1.57	1.50	1.16
Inhibited communication	1.95	2.12	2.30	1.43	1.39	1.32
Submissive-dependent	1.53	1.74	1.44	1.89	1.78	1.58
Family attachment	2.59	2.93	2.17	2.78	2.53	2.54
Anxious rumination	1.82	2.17	1.98	1.96	1.94	1.61

*0 = not at all; 1 = extremely

**1 = not at all; 5 = extremely

***1 = functioning well; 5 = extremely maladjusted

255

TABLE 73a

Frequency of Scaled Scores
of Hospice Patients

	Hospice Patients					
			N = 39			Missing
	1	2	3	4	5	Value
From SCL-90						
Somatization	8	24	2	1	0	4
Interpers. sensitiv.	26	8	1	0	0	4
Depression	8	15	11	1	0	4
Anxiety	17	14	3	1	0	4
Hostility	24	10	1	0	0	4
						Missing/
	1	2	3	4	5	N.A.
From SAS-SR						
Work outside the home	1	0	0	0	6	32
Work at home as a housewife	0	3	12	4	1	19
Social & leisure activ.	1	20	12	0	0	6
Relationship with extended family	11	20	2	0	0	6
Relationship w/spouse	1	16	7	0	0	15
Fulfillment of parental role	4	7	0	0	0	28
Functioning within family unit	12	13	2	2	0	10
Enough money to care for own & family's financial need	26	2	1	1	3	6
Performance at work	1	0	0	0	6	32
Friction	27	6	0	0	0	6
Inhibited communicat.	3	26	3	1	0	6
Submissive-dependent	7	11	12	8	1	0
Family attachment	3	13	10	4	3	6
Anxious rumination	5	18	9	1	0	6

NOTE: Each cell of the table contains a number that represents the number of patients in the designated study group whose mean score on the

TABLE 73b

Frequency of Scaled Scores
of Non-Hospice Patients

| | Non-Hospice Patients | | | | | |
| | | N = 35 | | | Missing | |
	1	2	3	4	5	Value
From SCL-90						
Somatization	2	17	12	4	0	0
Interpers. sensitiv.	11	9	11	4	0	0
Depression	1	9	16	9	0	0
Anxiety	6	11	10	7	1	0
Hostility	11	13	5	5	1	0
						Missing/
	1	2	3	4	5	N.A.
From SAS-SR						
Work outside the home	0	0	0	0	4	31
Work at home as a housewife	0	2	15	3	0	13
Social & leisure activ.	0	15	9	1	0	0
Relationship with extended family	9	18	6	2	0	0
Relationship w/spouse	1	13	12	2	0	7
Fulfillment of parental role	2	6	2	0	0	25
Functioning within family unit	6	15	8	5	1	0
Enough money to care for own & family's financial need	24	8	1	0	0	2
Performance at work	0	0	0	0	4	31
Friction	10	19	5	1	0	0
Inhibited communicat.	2	22	8	3	0	0
Submissive-dependent	8	10	15	2	0	0
Family attachment	1	8	16	9	1	0
Anxious rumination	2	17	13	3	0	0

composite variable in question rounds off to the
integer listed above.
  N.A. = Not Applicable.

TABLE 74 a

Frequency of Scaled Scores of
Hospice Primary Care Persons

	Hospice Primary Care Persons					
	1	2	3	N = 39 4	5	Missing Value
From SCL-90						
Somatization	22	15	1	–	–	1
Interpers. sensitiv.	25	10	3	–	–	1
Depression	12	18	7	1	–	1
Anxiety	18	16	3	1	–	1
Hostility	20	15	2	1	–	1
	1	2	3	4	5	Miss'g/ N.A.
From SAS-SR						
Work outside the home	9	6	1	–	6	17
Work at home as a housewife	11	10	4	–	–	14
Social & leisure activ	3	28	7	–	–	1
Relationship with extended family	16	17	4	–	–	2
Relationship w/spouse	6	22	5	–	1	5
Fulfillment of parental role	8	8	3	–	–	20
Functioning within family unit	12	16	5	1	1	4
Enough money to care for own & family's financial need	21	10	4	1	2	1
Performance at work	7	7	1	1	6	17
Friction	22	14	2	–	–	1
Inhibited communicat.	12	20	5	1	–	1
Submissive-dependent	1	16	19	3	–	–
Family attachment	6	21	10	1	–	1
Anxious rumination	10	23	4	1	–	1

NOTES:

Each cell of the table contains a number that represents the number of primary care persons in the designated study group whose mean score on

TABLE 74b

Frequency of Scaled Scores of
Non-Hospice Primary Care Persons

	Non-Hospice Primary Care Persons					
	N = 35					Missing
	|1|	2|	3|	4|	5|	Value |
From SCL-90						
Somatization	8	18	5	4	-	-
Interpers. sensitiv.	9	16	8	2	-	-
Depression	-	14	15	5	1	-
Anxiety	3	15	11	6	-	-
Hostility	9	11	9	5	1	-

						Miss'g/
	|1|	2|	3|	4|	5|	N.A. |
From SAS-SR						
Work outside the home	1	8	6	1	3	16
Work at home as a housewife	1	7	12	4	-	11
Social & leisure activ	1	13	18	3	-	-
Relationship with extended family	6	21	7	1	-	-
Relationship w/spouse	-	17	14	-	1	3
Fulfillment of parental role	2	7	5	-	-	21
Functioning within family unit	3	20	12	-	-	-
Enough money to care for own & family's financial needs	19	10	1	3	1	1
Performance at work	1	6	6	3	3	16
Friction	4	21	9	1	-	-
Inhibited communicat.	2	18	13	2	-	-
Submissive-dependent	6	17	10	2	-	-
Family attachment	2	18	10	5	-	-
Anxious rumination	1	17	15	2	-	-

the composite variable in question rounds off to
the integer listed above.

N.A. = Not applicable.

TABLE 75

Summary of Differences Between Hospice and Non-Hospice Patients and Primary Care Persons on Psychosocial Scores as Detected by the Independent T-Test, the Paired T-Test, and the Sign Test

	Hospice Patients Compared with Non-Hospice Patients			Hospice Primary Care Persons Compared with Non-Hospice Primary Care Persons		
	Independent T-Test	Paired T-Test	Sign Test	Independent T-Test	Paired T-Test	Sign Test
From Zuckerman*						
Anxiety	< .01	< .01	< .01	< .01	< .01	< .01
Depression	NS	NS	< .05	< .01	< .05	< .01
Hostility	< .01	< .05	< .01	< .01	< .01	< .01
From SCI-90*						
Somatization	< .01	< .01	< .01	< .01	< .01	< .01
Interpersonal sensitivity	< .01	< .01	< .01	< .01	NS	< .01
Depression	< .01	< .01	< .01	< .01	< .01	< .01
Anxiety	< .01	< .01	< .01	< .01	< .01	< .01
Hostility	< .01	< .01	< .01	< .01	< .01	< .01

(continued)

Table 75 - continued

From SAS-SR [***]

Mean social adjust. score	NS	NS	< .01	< .01	< .01
Work outside the home	**NS**	–	**NS**	NS	**NS**
Work at home as a housewife	NS	NS	< .01	< .01	< .01
Social & liisure activ.	< .01	< .05	< .01	< .01	< .01
Relationship w/extended family	< .01	< .05	< .01	< .01	< .01
Relationship w/spouse	< .05	**NS**	< .01	< .01	< .01
Fulfillment of parental ro.	NS	NS	< .05	**NS**	< .01
Functioning within family unit	< .01	< .01	< .05	< .05	< .01
Enough money to care for own & fam's financ. need	NS	NS	**NS**	**NS**	**NS**
Performance at work	NS	NS	< .01	< .01	< .05
Friction	< .01	< .01	< .01	< .01	< .01
Inhibited communication	NS	NS	< .01	< .05	< .01
Submissive-dependent	< .01	< .05	< .01	< .01	< .01
Family attachment	NS	NS	< .01	**NS**	< .01
Anxious rumination	< .05	NS	< .01	< .01	< .01

261

[*] 0 = not at all; 1 = extremely
[**] 1 = not at all; 5 = extremely
[***] 1 = functioning well; 5 = extremely maladjusted

1.   Campbell and Stanley, <u>Experimental</u> <u>and</u>
<u>Quasi-Experimental</u> <u>Designs</u> <u>for</u> <u>Research</u>
(Chicago: Rand-McNally Co., 1963), p. 12.

2.   L. R. Derogatis, SCL-90 Administration,
Scoring and Procedures Manual - I.

3.   Myrna M. Weissman and Sally Bothwell,
"Assessment of Social Adjustment by Patient
Self-Report," <u>Archives of General Psychiatry</u>,
Vol. 33, Sept. 1976, pp. 1114-1115.

4.   Bernard Lubin, "Adjective Checklists for
Measurement of Depression," <u>Archives of General</u>
<u>Psychiatry</u>, Vol. 12, January 1965, pp. 57-62.

5.   Derogatis, SCL-90 Administration.

6.   Lubin, "Adjective Checklists."

7.   Weissman and Bothwell, "Assessment of Social
Adjustment."

8.   A multipoint variation of the Kuder-
Richardson 20 formula known as coefficeent alpha
was the particular measure used by Derogatis in
calculating the internal consistency for the
nine measures of the SCL-90 from the data of
two hundred nineteen volunteers (L. R.
Derogatis, SCL-90 Administration, Scoring and
Proceduees Manual - I, p. 33). The approach
involved treating the within-form correlations
among the items as analogous of correlations
between alternate forms, and assumed that the
average correlation among existing items would
be equivalent to the correlation among items
comprising the hypothetical alternative form.
The entire set of coefficients yielded was
indicative of satisfactory consistency and
ranged from a low of 0.77 for psychoticism to
a high of 0.90 for depression.

9.   Derogatis, SCL-90 Administration, p. 340.

10.   Bernard Lubin, "Fourteen Brief Depression
Adjective Checklists," <u>Archives of General</u>

Psychiatry, Vol. 15, August 1966, pp. 205-208.
11. Lubin, "Adjective Checklists."
12. Derogatis, Rickles and Rock detected a high degree of concurrent criterion-oriented validity in contrasting the dimension scores of the SCL-90 with scores from the Minnesota Multiphasic Personality Inventory (MMPI). Convergence was also detected in a study of Bololoucky and Horvath which correlated like symptom dimensions of the SCL-90 and the Middlesex Hospital Questionnaire. A number of other studies have examined the ability of the SCL-90 to provide clinical discrimination of importance to the validation process. Derogatis and Cleary have studied the degree of confirmation of the hypo-thesized internal structure of the instrument by empirically based analyses. Their data and information from other studies suggest that the hypothetical symptom constructs of the SCL-90 may be distilled from clinical data, and demonstrate that their empirical measures correlate well with established and accepted external criterion measures. Derogatis, SCL-90 Administration.
13. Lubin, "Adjective Checklists," p. 61.
14. S. R. Hathaway and J. C. McKinley, "Minnesota Multiphasic Personality Inventory" (Manuel, New York: Psychological Corp,, 1951).
15. A. T. Beck et al., "Inventory for Measuring Depression," _Archives of General Psychiatry_, Vol. VI, August 1961, pp. 561-571.
16. Lubin, "Fourteen Brief Checklists," pp. 205-208.
17. Weissman and Bothwell, "Assessment of Social Adjustment."
18. Jum C. Nunnally, _Psychometric Theory_ (New York: McGraw-Hill Company, 1967), pp. 172-235.
19. Lee J. Cronbach, _Essentials of Psychological Testing_ (Revised) (New York: Harper & Row, 1960).
20. Sidney Siegel, _Nonparametric Statistics for the Behavioral Sciences_ (New York: McGraw-Hill

Book Co., 1956), pp. 68-75.
21. M. Zborowski, "Cultural Components in Responses to Pain," Journal of Social Issues, 8 (1952), 16-30.

CHAPTER 11

Findings

All three statistical tests indicated that
Hospice patients and primary care persons
experienced significantly less anxiety,
depression, hostility, somatization, friction,
submission, and dependence than non-Hospice
patients and primary care persons (see tables
71-75). The three tests also unanimously
reported that Hospice patients and primary care
persons experienced greater satisfaction in
their social and leisure activities and in
their relationships with their extended
families than did non-Hospice patients and
primary care persons. On all three instruments
Hospice patients reported better functioning
within the family unit and less interpersonal
sensitivity than non-Hospice patients. Hospice
primary care persons reported better overall

social adjustment, more satisfaction in housework, better marital relations, and less
inhibited communication than non-Hospice primary
care persons.

Differences between the Hospice and non-
Hospice groups on psychosocial scores, as
determined by the three statistical tests used
in the analysis of the data have been
summarized in Table 75. The results of the
independent t-test were identical to the
results of the paired t-test with a few exceptions: The independent t-test indicated
significant differences between the Hospice and
non-Hospice groups with respect to anxious
rumination and marital relationships of patients,
and interpersonal sensitivity and family relations of primary care persons (fulfillment of
parental role, functioning within the family
unit, and excessive dependence on one's family),
whereas the paired t-test did not. The sign
test, like the independent t-test, detected
differences between the Hospice and non-Hospice
study groups with respect to the anxious
rumination and marital relationships of
patients, and the interpersonal sensitivity and
family relations of primary care persons, which
the paired t-test did not detect. The sign
test also recorded significant differences in
depression, work performance and family attachment of Hospice versus non-Hospice patients
which were not indicated by either the paired
t-test or the independent t-test.

The stresses and symptoms that were most
problematic for Hospice and non-Hospice
patients alike, as indicated by higher mean
scores, were anxiety and depression, feelings
of submission, dependence, and excessive
attachment to family, and relating to one's
spouse. According to the results of sign tests

266

and t-tests, these were among the items most
significantly affected by Hospice care. Female
Hospice patients scored significantly lower than
female non-Hospice patients on 17 of the 23
maladjustment variables measured in the study.
Anxiety, depression, hostility, somatization,
interpersonal sensitivity, and several aspects
of social adjustment were more problematic for
non-Hospice than for Hospice female patients.
Scores of male Hospice patients were significantly lower than those of male non-Hospice
patients on only seven variables; all other
differences between the two male patient groups
were not significant. Similarly, patients of
high socioeconomic status were significantly
different with respect to only one variable,
whereas Hospice patients of low socioeconomic
status showed significantly lower levels of
maladjustment than non-Hospice patients of the
same class background on 18 of 23 variables.
Such marked differences across sex and socioeconomic status regarding the effectiveness of
Hospice care warrant further investigation and
may prove helpful in isolating a target population for the most effective delivery of Hospice
services.

Primary care persons of both Hospice and
non-Hospice origin experienced more friction
with people around them than did patients from
the respective study groups. Primary care
persons were, in general, also more hostile and
less anxious and depressed than patients. The
extent to which primary care persons were found
to somatize their problems was surprisingly
high, although not quite as high as among
patients. Hospice primary care persons
exhibited significantly lower levels of
maladjustment on 22 of the 23 variables
measured according to results of the sign test

and on 21 of the 23 variables measured according to the results of the t-test. <u>Thus, more significant differences were observed among primary care persons than among patients; Hospice services presumably had a greater effect on primary care persons than on patients.</u> This surprising and important finding points to important benefits of Hospice care and should be considered in future research.

In the Hospice group, female primary care persons were troubled less by anxiety, depression, hostility, somatization, inter-personal sensitivity, and several aspects of social adjustment than were non-Hospice female primary care persons. Male primary care persons in the Hospice group differed significantly from male non-Hospice primary care persons only with respect to anxiety and depression. The hostility scores of primary care persons of high socioeconomic status were significantly different, as were those of primary care persons from the lower socioeconomic classes. Hospice primary care persons of lower socioeconomic status demonstrated lower scores in somatization, interpersonal sensitivity, and overall social adjustment than Hospice primary care persons of higher socioeconomic status. However, inter-pretation of these results must be tempered by an awareness of the circumstances and problems involved in conducting such a study with terminally ill patients, such as problems of external validity and sampling variation. In particular, between-group differences in actual survival time (as distinct from assigned prognosis) may reflect differences in the stages of psychological adjustment the patient has passed through at the time of the self-report consult.

It is estimated that non-Hospice patients spent 50 percent more time in either an acute-care hospital or some other institutional setting than Hospice patients. Non-Hospice patients were channeled in and out of hospitals to a greater extent than were Hospice patients and as a consequence spent less time living with their families. Few patients in the non-Hospice study group received any form of home care. A strong possibility exists, therefore, that home care, not Hospice service, was the critical element in alleviating the problems of terminal illness for Hospice patients and their families. However, if this is true, the fact remains that Hospice has presented itself as an effective vehicle for such home care assistance. Further study is required to determine which elements of Hospice care are specifically responsible for improvements detected in the Hospice group.

According to the subjective assessment of the data gatherer, non-Hospice patients experienced more pain than Hospice patients. The lower pain levels of Hospice patients are consistent with the results of studies by Lamerton in which the pain of cancer patients at Saint Christopher's Hospice in London was significantly reduced by special efforts at pain control. Lamerton has posited that the pain experienced by those being cared for at home could be markedly reduced by introducing a Hospice home care team and outpatient clinic into the patient's total care regimen. Prolonged terminal suffering and the nightmare of chronic pain undoubtedly tend to sap an individual's vital energy, which would otherwise be utilized in coping with the tremendous emotional, spiritual, and practical burdens of dying. Indeed, emotional stress and anxiety are often provoked by anticipation of the cyclic return of pain. The possibility exists, therefore, that application of the Hospice philosophy of pain control contributed significantly to the

269

relative well-being reported by Hospice patients. The effect of proper pain control is a high priority item for subsequent research.

Whereas 72 percent of patients in the Hospice study group died at home, most of the control group patients have or will have died in a hospital. Perhaps the security of knowing one's last hours were to be spent in familiar surroundings among the closest of friends and loved ones was a major source of comfort to Hospice patients.

In contrast to non-Hospice patients, Hospice patients had access to immediate care on a 24-hour-per-day basis. Assistance to Hospice patients and primary care persons was as close as the telephone: either a clinician's call or a nursing care visit followed each request for help within 10 to 20 minutes. The security rendered by this mode of care contrasts with the situation faced by patients such as those in the non-Hospice study group, who elected to remain at home for the duration of their illness and, as a consequence, frequently found themselves isolated from the medical community.

Clinicians and nurses in acute-care facilities as well are usually unaccustomed to the problems of the chronically ill and a number of studies have indicated that the terminal cancer patient's physical distress is not adequately controlled in the general hospital setting. The control of minor or problematic symptoms may often be overlooked in the busy atmosphere of the acute-care hospital. Only a properly trained nurse or family member is aware of the significance and upset caused by such problems as dyspnea, diarrhea, and loss of appetite. Attention to such symptoms may have contributed to the significant difference in the responses of Hospice and non-Hospice patients to

the three study questionnaires. Lower levels of
anxiety and maladjustment may also be due at
least in part to the willingness of the Hospice
staff to deal with the emotional needs that
influence a patient's perception of pain.
Because of general avoidance of dying perients
by other health care personnel, treatment of the
emotional dimensions of pain is usually
neglected.

Summary

Although the trends in anxiety, depression,
hostility, and social adjustment recorded in the
study are enlightening in that they characterize
the nature and extent of specific problems
experienced by the two groups of patients and
primary care persons, the findings of the study
are limited and must be reviewed with caution and
an awareness of the shortcomings of the study
design (discussed in the previous chapter).

A necessary condition for the inference of
a causal relationship between Hospice care and
the findings of the study is that no plausible
alternative explanation of the findings exists.
However, the findings may be attributed merely
to differences in the availability of home care
assistance. That is, the essential element in
the Hospice program may have been merely the
home care, and not necessarily the features
unique to Hospice. The differences observed may
have been due to the fact that home care was
seldom available to the control group.

Although the statistically significant
differences indicated by the results of the
t-test have been used as the basis for conjecture
on the existence of effects of Hospice care,
such inferences should only be considered
tentative, given the nature of the data. No
statistical tests can compensate for a design

271

in which nonequivalent and nonrandomized groups receive different treatments.

It is therefore imperative that the findings of the present study be thoroughly explored. Those findings, although provisional, should be regarded as an initial step in the process of expanding the limited substantive knowledge of dying patients and their families. The major findings are listed below.

1. Anxiety, depression, relating to one's spouse, and feelings of submission were problems for both Hospice and non-Hospice patients.

2. Hospice patients had lower levels of anxiety, depression, and hostility than did non-Hospice patients.

3. Hospice primary care persons had lower levels of anxiety, depression, hostility, and many aspects of social maladjustment than did non-Hospice primary care persons.

4. In general, differences were more marked for women than for men and more marked in lower socioeconomic groups than higher socioeconomic groups.

5. In general, the differences ("benefits") appeared to be greater for the primary care persons than for the patients themselves.

Future progress in the field of terminal care will be contingent upon the accumulation of valid and reliable research data. Any

272

factors such as those isolated in the present study which potentially contribute to better terminal care should be thoroughly explored. Knowledge of the needs of the dying is essential to the determination of the manner in which those needs can best be met.

Despite the practical problems of obtaining a randomized, representative sample of adequate size for a more rigorous study in a terminal care setting, it is clear that such a study would provide information of great value to the Hospice movement as well as to those in the field of death and dying. It is hoped that the current project will serve as an incentive for more conclusive subsequent studies of terminally ill patients and their families.

Selected Bibliography

Buckingham, R.W., and S.F. Filey. "A Guide to Evaluation Research in Terminal Care programs." Journal of Death Education, June 1978:127-141.

Buckingham, R.W.; S.A. Lack; et al. "Living with the Dying: Use of the Technique of Participant Observation." Canadian Medical Association Journal 115 (December 18, 1976): 1211-15.

Carey, R.J. "Living Until Death." Hospital Progress 55, no. 2 (February 1974):82-87.

Crase, Dixie, and Darrell Crase. "Live Issues Surrounding Death Education." Journal of School of Health, February 1974:70-73.

Davis, Kenneth. "Ergos, Thanatos: The Not-So-Benign Neglect, or Sexuality, Death and the Physician." Texas Reports on Biology and Medicine 32, no. 1 (Spring 1974):43-48.

Donabedian, Avidis. "Evaluating the Quality of Medical Care." A Guide to Medical Care Administration LL, American Public Health Association. Milbank Memorial Fund Quarterly 44, no. 2 (July 1966):166-203.

Elinson, J. "Effectiveness of Social Action Programs in Health and Welfare." Assessing the Effectiveness of Child Health Services, Report of the Fifty-Sixth Russ Conference on Pediatric Research. (977):79-88.

Feifel, H. New Meanings of Death. New York: McGraw Hill Book Co., 1978.

Feifel, H. "Perception of Death." Annals of
the New York Academy of Science 164 (1969):669.

Gerber, Irwin, et al. "Anticipatory Grief and
Aged Widows and Widowers." Journal of
Gerontology 30, no. 2 (1975):225-229.

Glick, I.O.; R.S. Weiss; and C.M. Parkes.
The First Year of Bereavement. New York:
J. Wiley and Sons, 1974.

Gorer, Geoffrey. Death, Grief and Mourning in
Contemporary Britain. London: Crosset, 1965.

Hackett, A., and M. Weisman. "Reactions to the
Imminence of Death." In Grosser, ed., The
Threat of Impending Disaster, Cambridge:
M.I.T. Press, 1964.

Hagen, E.D., and R.L. Thorndike. "Evaluation."
In Encyclopedia of Educational Research (3rd
ed.). New York: MacMillan, 1960:482-486.

Herzog, E. Some Guidelines for Evaluative
Research. Washington, D.C.: Government
Printing Office, 1959.

Hinton, John. "The Physical and Mental Distress
of the Dying." Quarterly Journal of Medicine
32 (1963):1.

_____. Dying. Baltimore: Penguin Books, 1974.

_____. "Talking with People about to Die."
British Medical Journal 3 (1974):25-27.

Holford, R.M. "Terminal Care." Nursing Times,
January 1973:113-115.

Janzen, Erica. "Relief of Pain." Nursing

Forum 13, no. 1 (1974).

Kahn, Sigmund B., and Vincent Zarro. "The Management of the Dying Patient." Seminars in Drug Treatment 3, no. 1 (Summer 1973):37-45.

Kelman, H.R., and J. Elinson. "Strategy and tactics of Evaluating a Large Scale Medical Program." Proceedings of the U.S. Social Statistics Section, Washington, D.C.: American Statistical Association (1968): 169-191.

Klinegerg, O. "The Problem of Evaluation Research." International Social Science Bulletin 7, no. 3 (1955):347-351.

Krant, Melvin J., and Lee C. Johnston. "An Evaluation of Existential Dimensions of Late-Stage Cancer Patients and Their Families. Boston: Unpublished Report from the Tufts Cancer Psychosocial Study Unit.

Kubler-Ross, Elisabeth. On Death and Dying. New York: MacMillan Co., 1969.

Lack, S.A. "Management of Pain in Terminal Cancer." Medical News-Tribune 4, no. 38 (September 18, 1972) 2, England.

_____. "I Want to Die While I'm Still Alive." Death Education 1 (1977):165-176.

_____. "Philosophy and Organization of a Hospice Program--Psychological Care of the Dying Patient." University of California School of Medicine, San Francisco, Charles A. Garfield (ed.), 1977.

Lack, S., and R. Lamerton. "The Hour of our

Death." Cassell and Collier, MacMillan Ltd., 1974.

Lamerton, R. "Teamwork." Nursing Times, December 1972: 1642-1643.

_____. "Care of the Dying, Pt. IV, The Pains of Death." Nursing Times 69 (January 1973).

_____. Care of the Dying (Priority Press Ltd., 1973).

LeShan, L. "The World of the Patient in Severe Pain of Long Duration." Journal of Chronic Disease 17, no. 119 (1974).

Lester, David, et al. "Attitudes of Nursing Students and Nursing Faculty Toward Death." Nursing Research 23, no. 1 (1974).

Marie Curie Memorial Foundation. "Joint National Cancer Surgery with the Queen's Institute of District Nursing." Report, 1952.

Melzack, R. The Puzzle of Pain. Harmondsworth, England: Penguin, 1973, 142.

Melzack, R., et al. "The Brompton Mixture: Effects on Pain in Cancer Patients." Canadian Medical Association Journal 115 (July 17, 1976):125-126.

Mount, B.M. "The Problem of Caring for the Dying in a General Hospital: The Palliative Care Unit as a Possible Solution." Canadian Medical Association Journal 115 (July 17, 1976):119-121.

_____. "Use of the Brompton Mixture in Treating the Chronic Pain of Malignant

Disease." Canadian Medical Association
Journal 115 (July 17, 1976):122-124.

Parkes, C.M. "The Emotional Impact of Cancer on
Patients and Their Families." Journal of
Laryngology and Otology 89, no. 12 (December
1975):1271-1279.

Porter, J.V. "A Therapeutic Community for the
Dying." Association of Operating Room Nurses
Journal 21, no. 5 (April 1975):838-843.

Rabin, D.L., and L.H. Rabin. "Consequences of
Death for Physicians, Nurses, and Hospitals."
In Brim et al., The Dying Patient, New York:
Russel Sage, 1970.

Rees, W. Dewi, and Sylvia G. Lutkins.
"Mortality of Bereavement." British Medical
Journal, October, 1967.

Rees, W. Dewi. "The Distress of Dying."
British Medical Journal 3 (1972).

Rose, Mary Ann. "Problems Families Face in Home
Care." American Journal of Nursing, March
1976:416-418.

Rosin, Arnold J.; Marcel Assael; and Leah
Wallach. "The Influence of Emotional Reaction
on the Course of Fatal Illness." Geriatrics,
July 1976:87-90.

Saunders, C.M. "The Nursing of Patients Dying
of Cancer." Nursing Times 55 (November 6,
1959):1091-1092.

_____. "The Care of the Terminal Stages of
Cancer." Annals of the Royal College of
Surgeons, Supplement to vol. 41 (1967).

_____. The Management of Terminal Illness.
London: Hospital Medicine Publications, 1967.

Shephard, David A. "Terminal Care: Towards An
Ideal." Canadian Medical Association Journal
115 (July 1976):97-98.

Twycross, R.G. "Clinical Experience with
Diamorphine in Advanced Malignant Disease."
International Journal of Clinical Pharmacol-
ogy, Therapy, and Toxicology 9, no. 3 (1974).

_____. "Diseases of the Central Nervous
System--Relief of Terminal Pain," British
Medical Journal 347 (1975):212-214.

_____. "Diamorphine and Cocaine Elixir
B.P.C. 1973." Pharm. Journal 212 (1974):153
and 159.

_____. "The Use of Narcotic Analgesics in
Terminal Illness." Journal of Medical Ethics
1 (1975):11-17.

_____. "The Use of Diamorphine in the
Management of Terminal Cancer." Journal of
Thanatology 2 (Summer-Fall 1972):733-743.

Twycross, R.G.; D.E. Fry; and P.D. Wills. "The
Alimentary Absorption of Diamorphine and
Morphine in Man as Indicated by Urinary
Excretion Studies." British Journal of
Clinical Pharmacology 1 (1974):491-494.

Weidman, A.D. On Dying and Denying: A Psychiatric Study of Terminality. New York:
Behavioral Pub. 1972.

Weiss, C. Evaluating Action Programs:
Readings in Social Action and Education.

Boston: Allyn and Bacon, 1972.

Williams, Robert L.; and Spurgeon Cole.
"Religiosity, General Anxiety, and Appre-
hension Concerning Death." Journal of Social
Psychology 75 (1968):111-117.

Worby, C.M.; and R. Babineau. "The Family
Interview: Helping Patient and Family Cope
with Metastatic Disease." Geriatrics (June
1974):83-94.

Worden, W.J. Personal Death Awareness.
Englewood, N.J.: Prentice Hall, 1976.

Yeaworth, Rosalee, et al. "Attitudes of Nursing
Students Toward the Dying Patient." Nursing
Research 23, no. 1 (1974):20-24.

Films

Lack, S.A. "Terminal Cancer: the Hospice
Approach to the Family." The Network for
Continuing Medical Education, 15 Columbus
Circle, New York, New York 10023, 1977.

_____. "Terminal Cancer: the Hospice
Approach to Pain Control." The Network for
Continuing Medical Education.